*For Beverly:
Best of luck;
Lynn*

Right Choices
An Insider's Guide to Selecting a Nursing Home

Published by Lynn Smith Enterprises

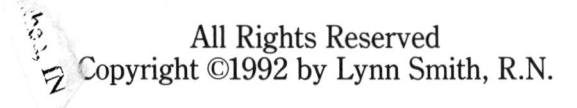

All Rights Reserved
Copyright ©1992 by Lynn Smith, R.N.

Library of Congress Catalog Card Number 92-24987

No part of this book may be reproduced or transmitted in any form or by any means, electronic or mechanical, including photocopying, recording or by any other information storage and retrieval system, without permission in writing from the author.

For information address:

Lynn Smith Enterprises
709 S. 18th St., #D
Lafayette, IN 47905

ISBN 0-9633706-0-X

Credits

Designated cartoons reprinted by permission of Thelma and Laura Canarecci from their book *Florence Nightingale Jones in Tender Loving Comedy*. Available from: Power Publications, 56 McArthur Avenue, Staten Island, N.Y. 10312 ($9.95 + $1.00).

Designated caricatures/cartoons reprinted by permission of E. Marsella Smith, R.N., M.S. Ed. from her book *The Geriatric Assistant*.

Designated caricatures created by Reneé Smith, an elementary school teacher, aerobics instructor, volunteer, and artist in addition to being a "sweetheart" of a daughter-in-law.

Cover design and designated cartoons and illustrations created by Gerry (G.T.) Murray, a freelance designer from the Lafayette, Indiana area.

Contents

Dedication and Acknowledgements............v
Special Acknowledgement for a Very
   Special Person, Bob Topping................ix
Foreword......................................xi
Preface......................................xiii
CHAPTER 1: As I See It......................1
CHAPTER 2: Before the Tour..................9

THE TOUR:
Exterior (1)................................11
Interior (2)................................12
Residents' Rooms (3).......................14
A Responsive Environment (4)...............16
Physical Plant (5).........................20
Dining Rooms (6)...........................21
Lounges (7)................................21
Staff Involvement (8)......................22
Patients'/Residents' Rights (9)............25
Adult Day Care (10)........................29
Restoration and Rehabilitation (11)........33
Observe the Resident (12)..................38
Resident Council (13)......................40
Dietary (14)...............................42
Spiritual Needs (15).......................46

Activities (16)	47
Financial (17)	53
CHAPTER 3: Residents' Rights and Advanced Directives	55
CHAPTER 4: Social History	65
CHAPTER 5: Psychotropic Medications and Restraints—Senility	69
CHAPTER 6: Positive Treatment Program	77
CHAPTER 7: Complaints and the Adjustment Period	83
CHAPTER 8: The Nursing Home Industry— A Bad Rap	87
CHAPTER 9: Predictions for the Industry	91
CHAPTER 10: Conclusion	95
Introspective Poem: *Don't Be Fooled By Me*	98
Suggested Readings	100
Letters from Nursing Home Staff Members	101
Visitation Check List	107

Dedication and Acknowledgements

All the many special people who touched my life so profoundly in some twenty years of being a part of the nursing home family.

The residents—Each one a wonderful, unique individual. Collectively, as a group, they had such a remarkable spirit of faith, trust and acceptance. Maybe it is as simple as their awareness and appreciation of the moment. For many, they had time to really smell the flowers, or the garlic, or the wine and savor it for its own beauty. For others, it was to look and really see the sunrise or sunset, to listen and really hear the birds, to feel the sun on their bodies with its warmth, or to sing a song with genuine joy. Individually, many gave love to us all. We as caregivers always need to remember that the residents need and want to give too. For many, it had been ages since anyone believed they had something worthwhile to give. In the taking and sharing of their love, we all became richer in the things that matter in life.

The families—Contrary to the sensationalized media opinion ("Granny dumping," for example), most I have known were caring and devoted to their loved ones.

There is an unwritten care law that links the care a person receives (wherever the person resides, home, hospital, nursing home, etc.) in direct proportion to the care, love and attention shown by the family. It is also true that many people without family (a resident in a nursing home for example) are "adopted" by a staff member, volunteer or special advocate. No question, the resident needs to feel this loving concern and support of family and friends. The family needs to be and remain involved in the entire process. The facility needs to seek and encourage that kind of participation and involvement. I want the families I was privileged to meet to know how much appreciation and respect I have for their dedication and devotion. Some of these same families also quietly and without fanfare "took into" their own families some of those residents who had no one.

The staff—I could write hundreds of pages about this group of unsung, underpaid saintly heroes we call the staff. These are the special people who reach out with an authentic, unconditional kind of tenderness and love. I refer not only to the professionals (nurses, social workers and therapists, etc.) but to the staff as a whole. Believe me, I had experience first hand that it doesn't take a college degree or worldly sophistication to be caring and attentive to all the little things. If space permitted, I could expound on thousands of such occurrences and occasions when a nurse's aide or a member of the housekeeping, dietary, secretarial, laundry or activity staff went quantum leaps beyond the "extra mile." I personally witnessed these special moments: when a nurse's aide prayed with a resident and stayed over on her own time to "be there;" when a housekeeper would bring a cup of hot chocolate to an early riser;

when a laundry employee mended clothes for a resident at home; and when a dietary employee baked a special treat on her own time because "the resident wanted it and it made her smile." The list is endless, but this is one way they can be publicly thanked, and I do *thank them* from the bottom of my heart.

Special thanks to Joan McIlwain, R.N., my partner and dear friend who shared these experiences with me and who has given me so much love and support in all things.

My sons: Tige (who is a recent law school grad "out to help the world be a better place") and Todd (who writes and sings beautiful music and still calls me Mama teasingly). They both independently read and re-read this book and gave me suggestions and encouragement.

My dear friend Mike, the father of Tige and Todd, who always encouraged me and believed in me unconditionally. His enthusiastic dedication to my commitment to and for the elderly enabled me to do what I have with the freedom to be me. I'm grateful for his abiding friendship.

My friend and typist and co-editor of this writing, Joan Vince. She has typed, re-typed and then once again—all with a smile and spirit of "We can do this." I couldn't have done it without her.

L.S.

Special Acknowledgement for a Very Special Person, Bob Topping

Bob's accomplishments include: Author of three books: 1. *The Hovde Years,* 2. *Century and Beyond,* 3. *The Book of Trustees of Purdue University.* He served at Purdue University as the director of the university news service, was the founder and editor of *Perspective* (an official university publication), assistant to the vice-president for development, and he retired as senior editor in the office of publications in 1990.

My heartfelt thanks, gratitude and appreciation to Bob who genuinely believes and practices unconditional giving to others. He willingly, joyfully and unselfishly offered his expertise in critiquing this book, as well as guiding me through every step of the publishing process.

When I first phoned him to ask a "few" questions, he was knee deep into the research for his commissioned book on the *History of Women at Purdue University.* In spite of his own pressing schedule, he immediately said he would be honored to read my book. Once he had the manuscript, in his "masters" hands, I felt such a sense of relief because I knew he would give me his honest analysis. Even as he was being interviewed on television about his new book, he had mine spread out in front of him. Because Bob is a writer by profession, I can only guess how many, many hours of his time and efforts went into the critiquing of this work.

When he first brought the book back to my office, he included a cover letter and left it in the door. I was so nervous, my hands shook as I read the first words of his letter: "This is great." I did a mental "Toyota jump," shed a few tears and called him to say thank you.

I have known Bob for many years and he is always the same genuinely caring person who reaches out to help others along the way. We had a motto at our nursing center for the staff and volunteers which said simply "IT IS A GOOD THING YOU DO." Bob, you exemplify that motto because I know, above all else, you wanted to see this book be available for others who may find it helpful in their time of need and anguish.

I want publicly to say to you "IT IS A GOOD THING *YOU* DO" and to sincerely thank you.

AN INSIDER'S GUIDE

Foreword

Lynn Smith is one of those rare and delightful persons who enriches the lives of everyone she meets. My good fortune was to meet her nearly a decade ago when she and Joan McIlwain owned and operated a nursing home and I desperately needed close care for my wife, stricken with what apparently was Alzheimer's Disease.

At my time of profound bewilderment, fear, and some hopelessness, I found Lynn and Joan, who not only offered a secure and loving environment for my wife, but reached out to me, calming my fears, refocusing my perspective, and offering me hope. Their shoulders were always there to cry on. They gave me strength to endure a tragedy that could have only one outcome for my wife: the blessed relief of a peaceful, dignified death.

Now Lynn has written a succinct, straightforward, even joyful book, the manuscript of which I was privileged to read and critique. Very early in my reading, the thought continued to repeat itself: I wish I had had this book when I was faced with the dilemma of finding a place that would meet my wife's needs better than I could.

More to the point, as I read Lynn's words, it became readily apparent that she felt compelled to set them down to articulate and summarize the comprehensive work, experience, and competence she has gained from three decades in the nursing profession. She knows all facets of the extended care milieu, having also been a "customer" of nursing home service when her own mother was a resident.

Beyond even that—at the risk of embarrassing her—I conclude that most of her motivation for writing this book comes simply from her enthusiastic concern for every living thing.

In this book, to all who may ever need the services of a nursing home for a loved one, Lynn Smith gives lucid insights that help one to make the "right" choices in making that crucial selection.

She also makes another point that can't be overemphasized: In any nursing home facility, the quality of care given your loved ones is always directly proportional to how much you demonstrate your own love and concern, and how often you provide them with regular face-to-face attention. Unconditionally true.

Lynn's generosity of spirit always brings comfort and a brighter outlook to all whose lives she touches, including those who will read her book.

So what more could any of us ask of a fellow human?

Bob Topping
1992

Preface

Some of what you read here will surprise you, some will startle you, but most of all, I want to help you, to reassure you of your options and your rights: *You* the *consumer, you* the family caregiver, *you* the *resident* or *prospective resident*. You really are in charge, like Invictus, *you* are the "Captain of your soul." I want this book to assist you to *take charge* and make an informed nursing home decision. You *can* and you *will* if you read these easy-to-follow guidelines and do your homework.

I waited to write this until now so as to avoid any potential conflict of interest, and to give myself enough years to take a good, hard look at the inside story. First, I'll give you a very brief synopsis of me and whence I come, and why I dare to write this kind of "how to" book. I am a registered nurse and a licensed nursing home administrator; and more importantly, I care. I care deeply about the care of people, especially the elderly. I went into nursing with rose-colored, idealistic values, and all the enthusiasm of a teenage cheerleader. I still feel that way about nursing and the care of people after thirty years of nursing. I have been involved in long term care for twenty plus years as a staff, hands-on nurse, a supervisor, a director of nurses, a patient care coordinator, former owner, president and CEO of a 145-bed healthcare center for eight years.

I should make all kinds of disclaimers, and I shall. I am a nurse, not a professional writer. I have volumes of notes and papers and letters from families and patients covering two tables in my house/office. Because of my personal experience and the desire to share it, I found myself trying to say it all. I kept getting off target, because to cover it all is impossible. Also, I was keenly aware of the people who will send me their own personal "horror" stories. I know I cannot correct these past "horrors," but I want very much for those to become isolated incidents and to assist you to deal with the here and now.

Obviously, I cannot speak for each and every nursing facility; I am certainly not an expert in the law of each state's regulations and problems. I can say, and I *do* say, that most nursing homes are good, and most of their staffs are among the most loving, devoted, caring, underpaid, and under-respected that you will find anywhere in the work place. More about the staff and how to relate to them later.

I will also say that all nursing homes are *not* created alike. Like any other industry, the few rotten apples spoil the reputation of all. There are still some private, locally owned facilities, but most are chains (a group of facilities under common ownership). Some are excellent, some are good, some are mediocre, some are poor. Some are drab and institutional, some are gorgeous in design and refreshingly warm and alive. I have no brilliant answers as to why these differences occur. What I can and will attempt to do is to give you the tools and the insight on "how to" choose a preferred facility smartly. I want you to know *what* to look for, *why* you are looking for it, and *how* to get the royal treatment you deserve. My emphasis will be on the positives, because they comprise what has been my own personal experience in a very dramatic, fulfilling way. My knowledge is not necessarily from textbooks, but rather from years of experience in the field. I have heard your fears and your overwhelming sense of guilt so I want to move you close to the process, take you through it, and help you to establish direction, dimension, and understanding.

L.S.

If I Can Stop
One Heart from Breaking

If I can stop one heart from breaking,
    I shall not live in vain;
If I can ease one life the aching,
    Or cool one pain,
Or help one lonely person
    Into happiness again
I shall not live in vain.

                      Emily Dickinson

CHAPTER 1

As I See It

The hospital calls and tells you that your wife is going to be discharged tomorrow, or that your mother must go to a skilled care center for rehabilitation or to recuperate. Both patients require nursing home care, and suddenly your world collapses. You are faced with a major decision: Which healthcare facility should be chosen? If you get nothing else from this book, I hope it will convince you that you must pay attention, do your research, and know the various available facilities in your area *before* the crisis occurs. The worst of all scenarios is having to make a major judgment call in a last-minute crisis situation. So please—do your homework and be prepared.

The best way you can prepare is to visit people in healthcare facilities, and to volunteer if you are able. In other words, if you are already involved, you know what the facilities in your community are like; you are aware and have first-hand knowledge of what's available and how you feel about one or some.

One of the ads that I ran when I was co-owner of a facility stated: "We have worked hard to earn your

TRUST and our REPUTATION." By all means check with your physician, friends, community leaders, Area Agency on Aging, clergy, people who have been there, and listen to what they have to say. But—and this is an important "but"—you must do your own choosing after investigation and research and then rely heavily on your gut instincts. Your instincts have served you well throughout your life. Use them!

You need to get out and visit the facilities if you have not been to any previously; there is no way around that. People sometimes pay more attention to the purchase of a car or refrigerator than they do to the placement of someone in a healthcare center! They will pour over consumer reports and trek to six or seven appliance stores to buy a new refrigerator or washer. Some of these same people will call a nursing home and ask only for prices. We are talking *people* here—not appliances! When you test-drive a new car, you get behind the wheel and experience it, get a feel for it, and you don't buy it until you have tested several and feel right about your choice.

There's no question that the cost is important, but you must first visit several facilities and determine what's included in the price. Are you going to pay extra for laundry, for rehabilitation, for an exercise program? Please refer to Section 17—Financial.

Not unlike the best restaurants, truck stops, and hotels ("Look at all the cars there; it must be good!"), the nursing homes which are usually full, i.e., at capacity, are generally the best ones. Nursing homes are like any other business, including hospitals; they exist to provide a service, and they need you. Just hope they never forget that *their business is service.* Look at the two sets of words on this subject and think about them:

Nursing and Home, Health and Care. The facility should not look, feel or act like a factory, warehouse, or sterile institution.

I say unequivocally that most people who are in need of a nursing home are looking first and foremost for a *caring place* with an excellent reputation for nursing care; preferably a place that exudes warmth, comfort, and trust. One of the major concerns is... "My mother is well now...etc., but what if...she suffers a CVA (stroke), what if...she becomes increasingly disabled or dysfunctional...what if, etc.?"

These and all the other "what ifs" should be more easily laid to rest if you feel comfortable and at ease regarding your choice of a healthcare facility.

As statistics prove, there seems to be a glut of hospital beds, and in some areas surplus nursing home beds. I prefer the word accommodations but the fact remains, increased competition is better for you as a consumer. In some market areas, you can actually get a set of Gucci luggage or an electric wok for checking into this or that hospital. The competition is fierce.

Regarding nursing home decisions, an underlying prejudice seems to exist among some social service and agency people who use many negative and pessimistic phrases. I most despise "at risk of the nursing home" (meaning the person's present living arrangements and deteriorating physical or mental condition exposes the person to the probability of nursing home placement). That always sounds like a dreaded disease to be feared and avoided.

Perhaps the greater cruelty is to be and feel alone, isolated, and depressed. Perhaps the agencies should weigh the reality of the aloneness and slow stagnation of a four-walls confinement versus the companionship, stimulation, and treatment potential of the nursing home. Perhaps the isolation of being alone can produce a kind of "benign neglect" for the resident.

Statistics support the fact that the greatest number of people "at risk" are those living alone and isolated. For them the domino effect sometimes takes over: No reason to get dressed; no reason to cook and eat, in essence, no reason to live. Depression sets in, leading to increased confusion and disorientation from sensory deprivation. Some people insist upon remaining at home or in their apartment, as if that's the most important thing in the world—to stay in that apartment or home. That may be important, but why not consider a plan to go to a nursing facility to feel better, get stronger so you can get out of the Nightgown Syndrome, or receive therapy and specialized care so you can return home to enjoy *quality of life?* Let me re-emphasize: nearly every healthcare center provides rehabilitation, and the doors *do open* to take you back home—if you are able and choose to do so.

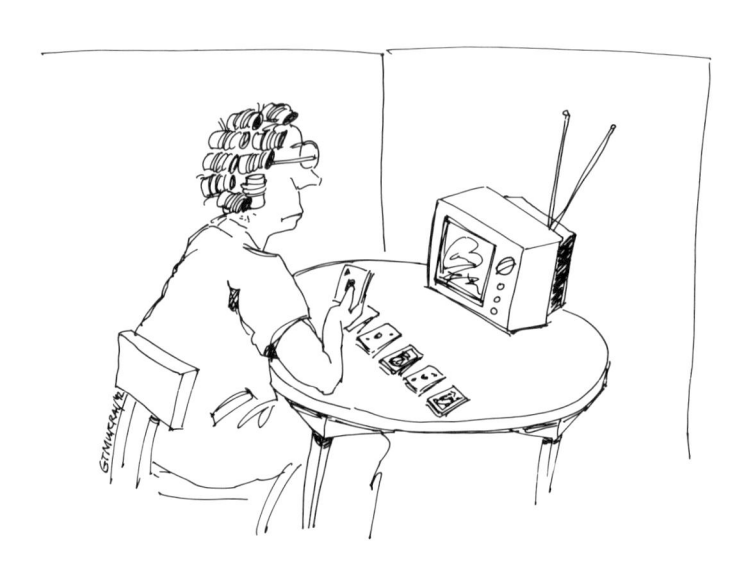

Several words of explanation about the Nightgown Syndrome: If you ever really want to get sick, the thing to do is to stay home and wear your nightie or pj's for three days. By the end of the three days, you will not only *feel* sick, and *act* sick, you'll *be* sick. Without the incentive to get up, get out and about and be active, we would all tend to disintegrate emotionally, with increased risk for physical problems as well. That's a fact. So please remember: The "at risk" of serious depression caused by deprivation of daily social contact and purpose in life is potentially far more dangerous to your loved one than any perceived disadvantage of being in a nursing facility.

Now the following statement may shock you: Many people like, yes, even *love* being in a healthcare center. In many cases, such is far preferable to the miserable loneliness, isolation, and boredom of being sequestered in an apartment. The following true story illustrates my premise. A wonderfully giving lady of eighty-seven who had been the volunteer chairman of the local hospital auxiliary for more than thirty years, and a dynamic force in the community for more than seventy years, gradually and unbeknown to anyone, had shut herself off from the world. She lived in a big, old house and became increasingly isolated. In retrospect it seems by her own account, she suffered from an underlying depression, and one thing led to another. Like a spiral, the depression led her to cease eating properly. She developed the Nightgown Syndrome. Soon her electrolytes (sodium, potassium, chloride) were out of balance and she became disoriented. Confusion took over her world. Fortunately a caseworker from her local Family Services Agency brought her to our nursing facility. The rest is history. For the first week she remained slightly confused and out of sync, but after eating proper foods, getting positive reinforcement with lots of TLC, and frequent reminders that people "needed" her help, she took over the place. I may just as well have gone on vacation. I loved watching her metamorphosis. It was exciting and exhilarating to see this lovely woman become alive and vibrant once again. Believe me, she took charge, and she spent her remaining years giving of herself, organizing us all, and spreading cheer and love to everyone. Such a wonderful way to live out one's life and how happy she was!

I am an advocate of the elderly; I was long before I owned a healthcare center. Yet, I must say the prejudice and negativism of many caring and well-meaning people often present serious negative connotations to the person trying to make an informed decision on health care. Often the nursing home becomes the proverbial "kick the can," because it seems that human nature requires a scapegoat and an outlet for anger and frustration over the entire process of aging. I hope this book at least causes those with such profound negativism to think in a more positive way about the better nursing facilities before inadvertently frightening people. If the decision is at hand, they are already frightened quite enough.

Many times "THE" (nursing) home becomes the scapegoat for underlying family problems. Some revolve around conflicts. The son thinks that his sister and her family should take mother into their home. The daughter would like very much to do just that, but she and her mother cannot live under one roof and still love each other the way they do now. Conflicts among siblings can become heated when they are trying to decide "what should be done with mother." Almost all the residents I knew (and I knew many well) did not, under any

As I See It 7

circumstance, want or desire to "live" with family—no way! What mother would want (and I know this from twenty plus years of listening) is to *take charge* of her own options and be treated in a respectful, caring manner, assuming she is competent and rational. She needs to be included in the "what to do" discussions and to assist in the decision-making process. You can't pitter-patter around the obvious. Come on out and say, "Mother, you are obviously getting worse...you are not eating...you have fallen four times in the past month...so we want to get you some help...some

A Family Conference

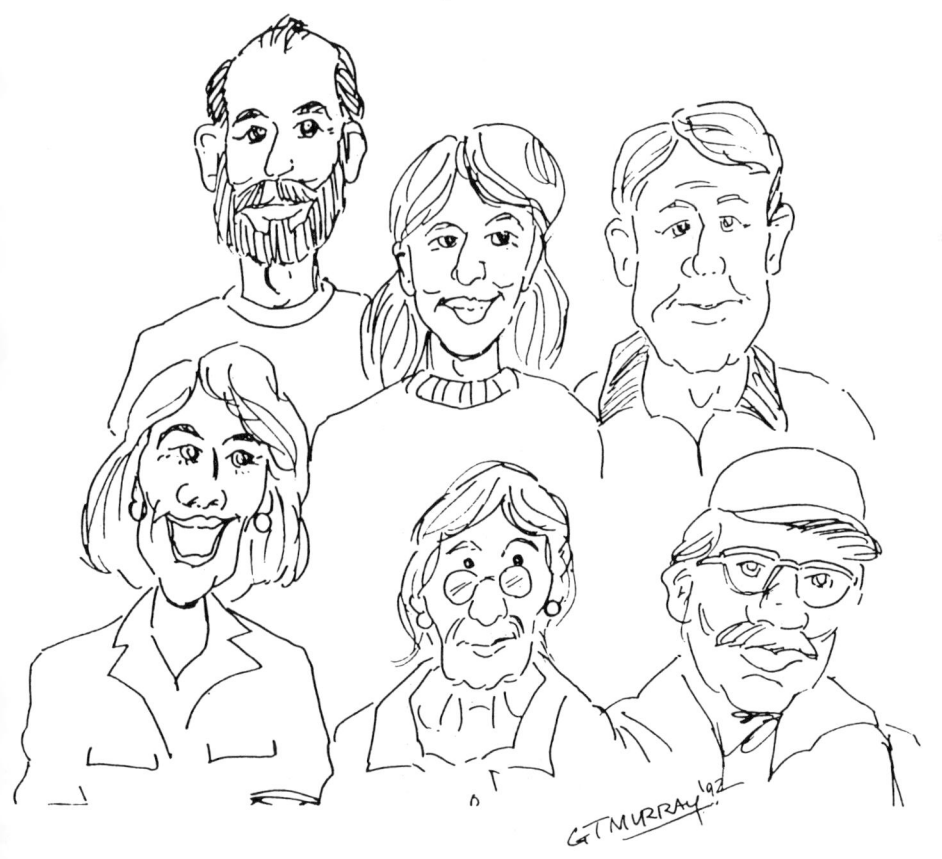

treatment." Please emphasize the treatment with the goal of feeling better—even of returning home if that's an option. Doors do swing out and open; they are not slammed shut. Statistics show that many people do, indeed, go home from nursing care centers. Talk in those terms and take mother to inspect a center if she is able. She probably only remembers the horror stuff and will be pleasantly surprised to see how things are being done today in a good facility. She may see some of her friends there and ask them how they feel about that particular place.

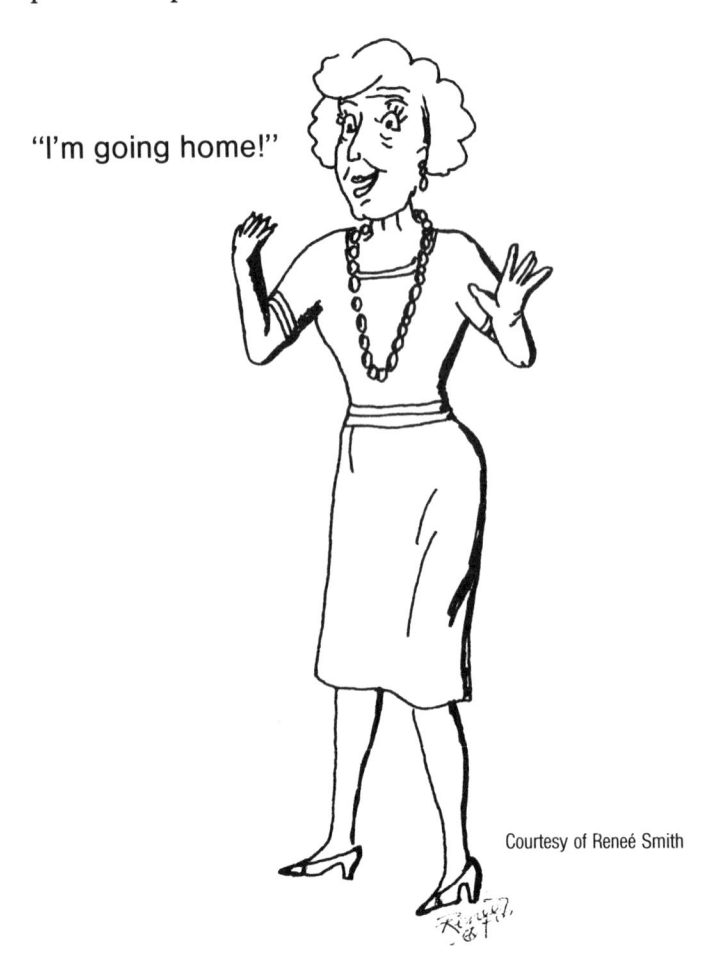

"I'm going home!"

Courtesy of Reneé Smith

CHAPTER 2

Before the Tour

The reality of the nursing home situation today is that all residents are not the same. All are in varying degrees of health and wellness. Some are quite sick, others on the road to recovery, and some are quite independent. Some are princes and princesses; some are darlings; some are wonderful, loving people who are dynamically involved with the world around them. Still others are just like people anywhere. There are those who grow old gracefully and with dignity, while others seem unapproachable, demanding, and yes, even grouchy and nasty at times.

With regard to those residents trying to relearn to feed themselves: it is not always a pleasant sight, but please do not fault the nursing home. Give its staff credit for promoting the rehabilitation process; that's the foundation of self-esteem. Once a person learns to get that spoon or fork back to the mouth following a stroke, for example, the sooner that person will feel better about himself and lead a more dignified existence with a sense of accomplishment. So as you are taking your tour of the facility pay attention to these kinds of things, and keep an open mind as to what's happening. It is not that they simply aren't bothering to feed Uncle Harry; it may be that they are simply trying to get Uncle Harry to do it for himself again.

Now, before you begin your tour of nursing homes, remember that all health care segments are vying for your business. Take a look at all of the nursing home advertisements that appear the next time your local newspaper features a special senior section. Remember five years ago when you were new in a community, and couldn't get in to see a physician? Now, however, you see signs in the doctor's office proclaiming "New Patients Welcome!" There has even been a resurgence of physician house calls. Thus, you can usually have the pick of the crop. *To choose carefully is to get the best accommodations.* It may be difficult and time-consuming, but it is well worth your effort.

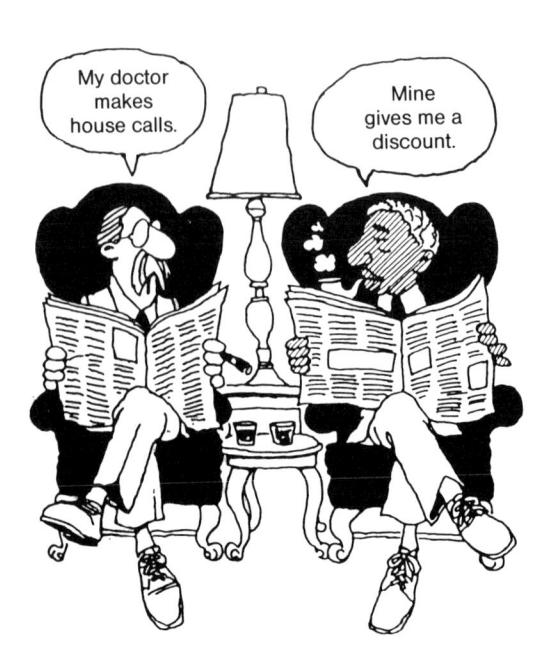

Before the Tour   **11**

A tear-out check list is included in the back of this book for your convenience. Detailed commentaries on some of the sections listed on the check list follow. By reviewing the check list before you tour, you can be sure to know just what to look for. Also, by reading the comments about each category, you will realize the importance of many features and be able to sort out those that have a high priority for your particular needs.

1. Exterior
Now is the time to take check list in hand and work through the agenda. I hope you will visit at least three facilities. When you arrive at the parking area, your first "curb appeal" impression will be of the grounds area. This is quite similar to the house-hunting process where your initial reaction sets the tone or stage for the place. If your senses are impressed with blooming flowers and a clean, well-manicured lawn, your first reaction is positive. Conversely, if the lawn is unkempt and littered with debris, you would need to question why. If there are no benches or lawn chairs—nothing happening outdoors, you should be concerned. Many facilities have a separate patio area with shaded spaces. It's my experience that nearly all nursing home residents enjoy the out-of-doors. Now maybe the weather is too hot, but that still doesn't excuse the fact that the lawn may be unkempt, and the fact that no one seems to be out there keeping the place neat and clean. The facility that cares generally shows it outside and in. Your *first impression* will be of great importance to the best of them, and with good reason. If it's winter, the parking lot should be clean and safe. For older, often disabled visitors, a driveway up to the door with a covered canopy is a real plus. Certainly special handicap parking and

adequate parking for visitors is a "must." If the American flag is flying at the front of the facility, that's a nice touch. If space permits, a vegetable garden for residents to dig in the earth is a much appreciated feature, especially in rural or outlying areas. Those who cannot actually work in the garden often enjoy planning for it and take pride in the harvest.

2. Interior

As you enter the facility, who greets you? Does a staff member transmit the facility's philosophy of caring and concern by asking, "May I help you?" Does it seem homey, warm, and welcoming? Or does it look and "feel" like an institution? Are the colors drab and hospital green or orange? Are there long corridors— stark and white? Or do you see pictures, art work/wall hangings, wallpaper and a sense of decor that is alive with color, texture and brightness?

Is it clean and polished? Do the floors sparkle?

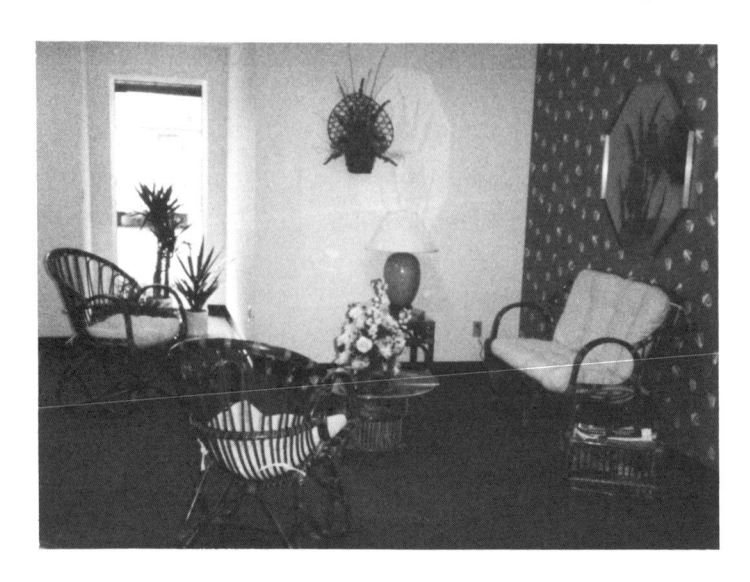

Before the Tour

Obviously, you should allow for inclement weather. If it's winter and there is ten feet of snow on the ground, the floors can't stay polished long once they've been tracked on. (Let's be fair.) Cleanliness *is* very important. I remember the warning given to a class by a Sister of Mercy while I was in nurses' training: "Don't you ever come on duty with dirty shoes—or I'm going to assume that your underwear is also dirty!" Now you can be sure that every student nurse who was instructed by that nun polished her shoes compulsively every night! So when you go into a facility, check to see if it is sparkling clean. Check how the facility manages infection control issues by observing good cleanliness practices (hand washing, the use of gloves, etc.).

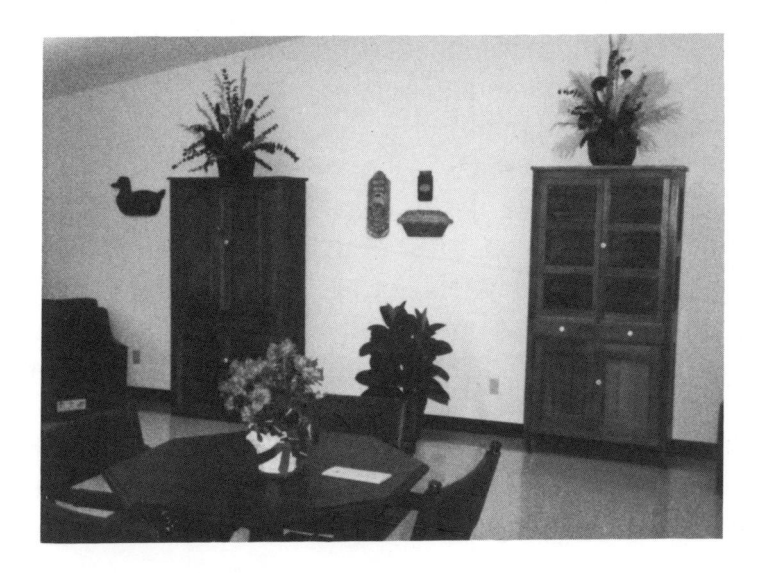

Next, look at the furniture. Is the furniture polished and clean? Look at the medical equipment such as wheelchairs and bedrails. Look at the bathrooms. Are they well lighted and ventilated? Are there mirrors? How can people look their best if the mirror/dressing area is out of scale or vision? Did an unpleasant aroma grab you the minute you entered? If so, that may spell trouble. Now, let me say this: There is a bumper sticker out there that says, "S--- Happens!" We've all seen that awful bumper sticker. I don't happen to like it, but let me tell you this, shocking as it may be, BMs do occur in nursing centers. People do go to the bathroom, people do have diarrhea sometimes, and some people are incontinent. So, as you pass down a hall and smell an isolated odor, give the facility a break. This is real. This is far preferable to the smell of an awful, flowery deodorant simply to cover up odors. After all, there are *real people living here*. The key phrase regarding odors is "pervasive versus isolated." What is your overall impression?

3. Residents' Rooms

The residents' rooms should be pleasantly furnished with color coordinated decor that is warm and pleasant. I hope each room is individualized and non-institutional in feel and appearance. Obviously, the room should be clean, fresh, and well lighted. The size of a double room is important to assure adequate private "territory" as well as the accommodation of special equipment such as wheelchairs and oxygen.

The rooms should also reflect the resident's personality with personal items: pictures of family; wall hangings; cards; a desk; a favorite chair from home; figurines, and so on. Most of us want our "stuff"—our treasures—around us. Have you ever noticed how almost everyone wants his or her wallet or purse? Even as my dad was dying and in severe pain, he repeatedly asked, "Is my wallet here?" I have seen this same concern shown for special possessions hundreds of times. "Stuff" can be thought of as therapeutic clutter and a collage of one's identity. You should be able to look at a room and see one's persona portrayed there. Resident rooms that have been personalized are a positive indication that people are the *number one* priority at the facility.

Watch for expressions such as, "We don't allow you to hang pictures here." To which I'd say, "Then I don't want to come here!" All that is required to hang a picture is a nail; eventually the facility will have to repaint anyway. You should be able to hang what you want in that room — within limits, of course. In my experience, some gentlemen had pictures they wanted to hang that exceeded common decency. When I was an administrator, I had to censor some pin-ups. You'd be surprised at how many older gentlemen read *Playboy*.

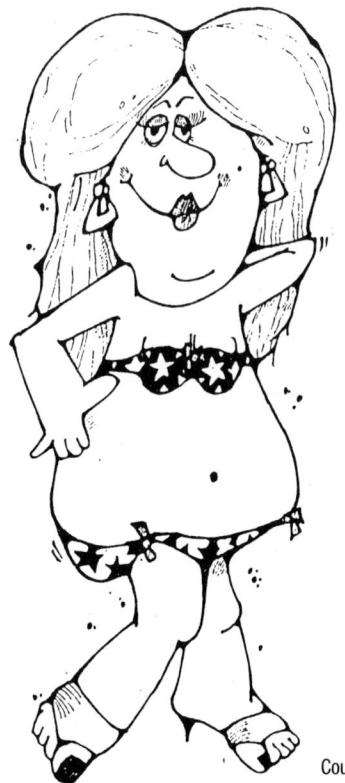

Courtesy of E. Marsella Smith

4. A Responsive Environment

Is it a lively, spirited place? Is it as user-friendly as your home? Are there pictures, plants, flowers? A cluttered "lived in" look is preferable to a sterile, institutional type atmosphere. Are people talking to one another? Are there conversation areas where people face each other? Do you observe clocks, calendars, and a sensory environment that is colorful and active? Are there bulletin boards, sign-up sheets for outings? Are appropriate seasonal reminders evident?

Please watch for the Tucked Into Bed Syndrome. If you observe that all the beds are made, and everyone is neatly "battened down" with sheets up to their heads, and the rooms are spotless with everything in place, I would ask, "Where are the people? Where is life? Is anything happening here?"

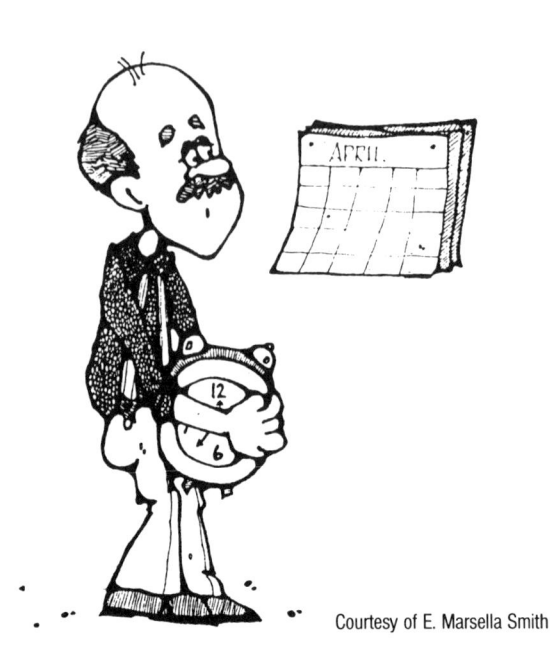

Courtesy of E. Marsella Smith

When we first took over the nursing home my partner and I had purchased, a policy existed that all beds had to be made by 11 a.m. What a mixed up priority. *People should always come first*—not beds. Well, the theory was that if someone came on a tour and saw that the beds were not made, they would think that the facility wasn't doing its job. Now, if I were shopping, as I've had to do for my own mother (I've also been a consumer) I would be far more concerned about looking at the people than at the beds.

Be aware of the Glittering Chandelier Syndrome that can blind you to the important issue which is *caring for and about people.* You can't always see it, but you can "feel" it and sense the love and trust. This caring *commitment* to people is what should dazzle you—not the pretty chandelier! Are the residents up and dressed

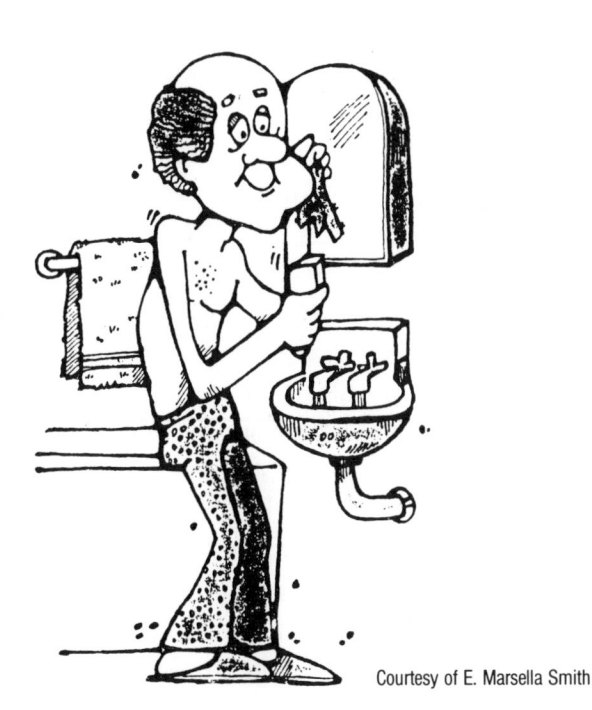

Courtesy of E. Marsella Smith

appropriately? At our center some men wore ties every day, several men wore coveralls, and some members of both sexes wore sweatsuits and sneakers. Most all of the women had their hair done at the in-house beauty salon. Some had their nails manicured and wore make-up and jewelry; they dressed socially for special occasions. Of course, dress should be based on resident preference and comfort. Will the residents' preferences be encouraged? Or will rules prevail? Is there a lights-out-at-8 p.m. mentality? I remember a kidney dialysis patient who was dying—a real love of a lad. The registered dietitian and the staff begged, pleaded, and teased to try to get him to eat, all to no avail. He said that he wanted and had a taste for pizza with sausage no less! The nurses called the doctor and you guessed it—he got his pizza. People should be encouraged to do their own "thing"— to follow familiar routines—and to have access to the things that hold a special, personal significance.

A good nursing home has nothing to hide. If the staff person giving you the tour avoids showing any particular area to you, ask to see it. While touring with the administrator, try to determine whether any of the residents actually know who the administrator is. In all fairness, if the resident does not recognize the administrator, it could be because of poor lighting, failing eyesight or memory or perhaps confusion. However, if you hear, "We are all one big, happy family here, and we all know each other by our first names," a flag should go up, especially if none of the residents recognize this "family" person, or you hear a resident say, "Who is she? Haven't seen her before."

"All that glitters is not gold!" is a wonderful old adage. Frankly, I would prefer to place my mother in a three-bed room if that's all that's available, if it's in a facility about which I feel good and secure. I feel much better about one that is into *people service*—one that backs that with adequate staff, and one that seems homelike—than I do about a pretty, chandeliered, sterile place. Do not choose to impress your friends; choose for yourself or what your loved one would like.

Our nursing home did a stunning new wing in mauve/mint decor, wicker, art work, and big fluffy towels. It resembled a lovely hotel. Most loved it, but several residents sniffed, "Looks too fancy for me; I'd rather stay in my old room." Besides that they did not like the big, fluffy washcloths. They didn't fit in their hands or ears and they weren't used to them.

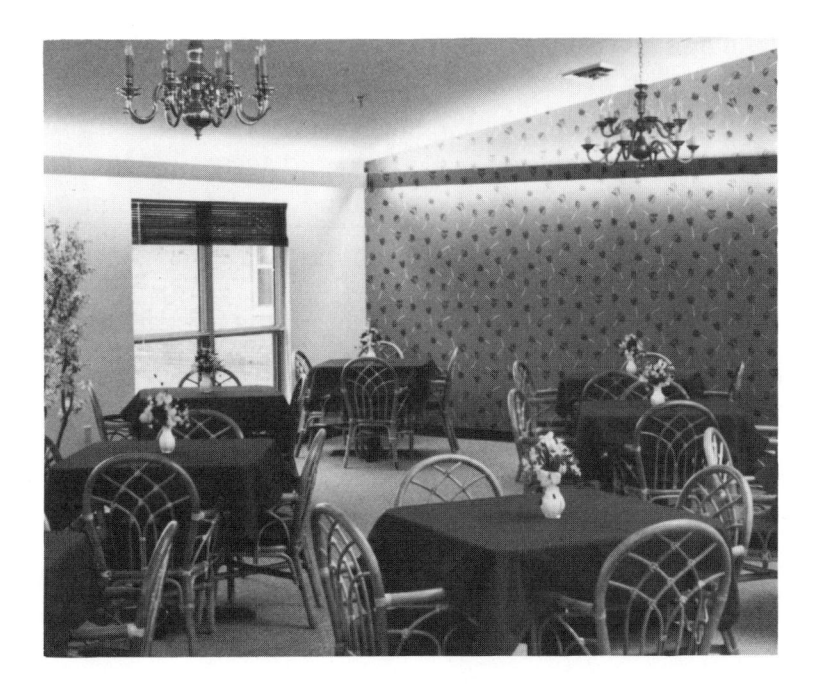

Something similar happened during our "Ethnic Food Days." Elegant, exotic food was served, but most preferred meat, potatoes, and pie—hearty Indiana fare—not fancy stuff, thank you. But at least all of these creative things provided stimulation and lots of conversation.

In our facility, there was an "emergency" resident council meeting called to advise the owners that they wanted their plain, "flimsy" washcloths back—*now!* Of course, they got them post haste! After all, the *residents should run the place* as though it's their home. Because it is.

5. Environment—Physical Plant

The home's physical environment must meet all applicable federal, state and local building and safety codes as well as OSHA (Occupational, Safety, and Health Administration) codes. Usually compliance and adherence to these standards are a "given" if the facility is to remain operational. However, should you want further detailed analyses regarding fire, tornado, and/or earthquake precautions and plans, you may ask to see the facility's disaster plan. You should note the sprinkler system, fire extinguishers, door alarm systems, etc. You may also see a copy of the latest federal/state survey of the facility which must be posted and accessible to you.

There should be adequate and glare-free comfortable lighting within the control of the resident. Touch lamps are helpful for arthritic hands. Obviously, the call-for-help button should always be within reach of the resident. The corridors or hallways should have handrails and be uncluttered and functionally safe. I doubt that you will encounter throw rugs or slippery floors in any facility, because a resident could easily slip and fall on these.

Resident rooms are discussed in a separate section. Some residents may have a private phone installed in their rooms. However, there must be a public telephone that is accessible to wheelchair residents, and one that accommodates the hearing-impaired resident.

6. Dining Rooms

The dining room should be reflective of home—friendly, cheerful and pleasant. Meals represent a social time for conversation and get-togethers. Generally, there are tables set up for four; compatibility is crucial. The tables often are adorned with tablecloths, cloth napkins and fresh flowers—done in a colorful motif. People are served in a gracious manner. The dining room should be a pleasant area, large enough for easy access and departure. Usually the larger facilities have several dining rooms. For all you purists and idealists out there, please try to look at the reality of what can and sometimes does happen. A person suffers a stroke, and with therapy finally begins to feed him or herself again. It is not a pretty picture; actually you are seeing a person relearning hand-to-mouth coordination. So please—don't turn away in disgust, because these people are on their way to recovery, on their way to regaining independence and, most importantly, self-respect. Some facilities have a graduated kind of seating and dining arranged according to need. One dining area will serve those who need much assistance; another will include those who are semi-independent, and a third for those who are the most independent.

7. Lounges

The lounge area should look and feel "comfy-cozy," inviting you to sit down and feel at home. Are people conversing with each other? It should not be an institutional setting. If rows of chairs are lined up around the corner of the room, how can people communicate? Small conversational centers where people may have relaxed social visits, sharing with each other are best. There should be reading lamps and available, up-to-date reading material, some of which should feature large, easy-to-read print. There should be a TV area that can be converted from small group seating to a larger area for movie (VCR) viewing, special entertainment programs, church services, or other group gatherings.

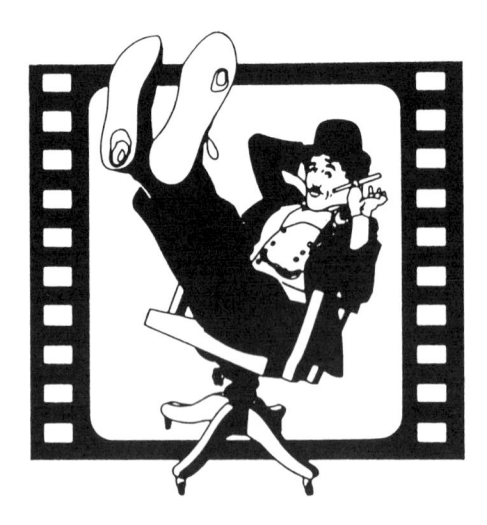

I believe strongly in humor therapy as well and the lounge can be used to view the classic movie comedies such as Red Skelton or Lucille Ball to tickle the funny bone and lighten the load.

8. Staff Involvement

Staff involvement is coordinated through the Care Plan meetings. Usually the charge nurse, social service director, registered dietitian, activity director—and any

Before the Tour

other caregiver directly involved with the resident—all meet to discuss and exchange information on the progress, or lack of improvement, and the objectives and methods for a particular resident's well-being. The resident and family members should be encouraged to attend these informal sessions. A resident and his or her family must feel safe and comfortable to speak freely and openly. After all, once again, note that the care of this *special person* is why each staff member is there. Please refer to the "Observe the Resident" chapter because it will refresh and assist you in your overall assessment of staff involvement.

You will encounter many staff members on your tour; undoubtedly you will be introduced to some. The best facilities are acutely sensitive to the level of your perception of them, especially as it correlates to your observation of the attitudes and behaviors of staff members who give direct care to the residents. As you know, people choose a restaurant for tasty food and friendly ambience. A healthcare facility, too, will be chosen for how it cares *for,* as well as *about,* its residents.

Facilities that practice this "trickle-down" philosophy take care of their staff with benefits, incentives, educational and motivational programs, and recognition of outstanding performance. You may see staff members wearing "I CARE" buttons, or perhaps you'll observe "Outstanding Employee" plaques on the walls.

An ideal or model staff will be involved and responsive to the residents. For example, you will hear the professional nurses or nursing assistants say, "How are you?" to a resident and *wait* for a response. You will see them make eye contact and bend over (if the resident is seated in a wheelchair) to show genuine concern and interest in the response. Most staff members know their residents well, and treasure and value each one as a special individual.

You will be able to feel this intrinsic goodness of the heart from many of the staff, because it is genuine. Many of these people whether in nursing, dietary, laundry, housekeeping, or activity jobs could earn more money in factory settings, but they love what they do—and it shows. You will note that most are caring, cheerful and enthusiastic. I have been privileged to know some of the "cream of the crop," and I cherish those wonderful memories. I could write pages of examples, but I will refer you to several essays written by some of these care providers beginning on page 101. You may read them yourself.

The staff should also be clean, groomed, and follow a decent, respectful dress code. Staff members are not permitted to use foul or offensive language. Remember: this population of adults is unaccustomed to the more commonplace four-letter words used today. Many still believe the word "gay" means happy or outgoing, as "he was a gay blade." Still, many others are in the know. As my own mother tells me: "I learn a lot from the TV talk shows; I know all about that stuff!"

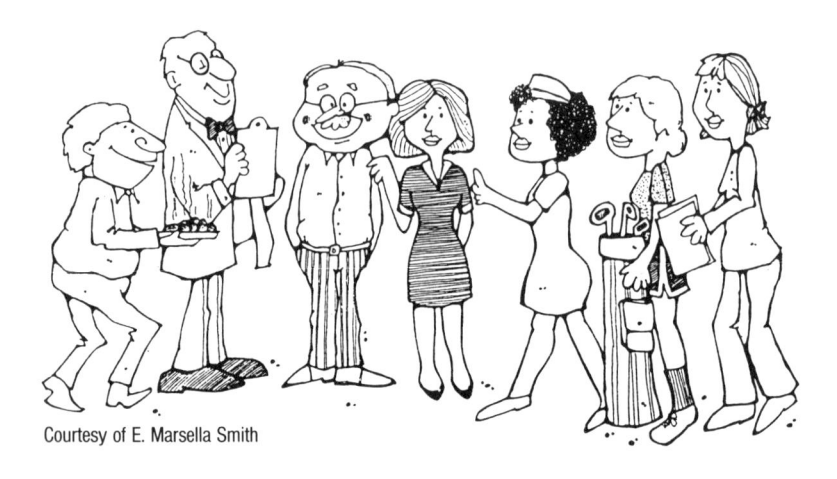

Courtesy of E. Marsella Smith

Staff members in a nursing home really function as an extended family and they have strong feelings about "their own." Most of us in this field really resent the stereotypical myth that says older people are depressing, complaining, crotchety, senile, or incapable of learning. It's just not true. We ought to know because we have experienced the wonderful ways in which one person can make a difference in another's quality of life. We know about the good stuff that goes on.

In all candor, no one facility is absolutely perfect on all counts. Because this is a people service industry, there are bound to be some flaws, some blemishes, some unfinished goals to achieve. The best facilities always seek new ways and means to strive for higher levels of excellence.

To paraphrase, "If the staff ain't happy, ain't nobody happy!" I've already discussed how the best facilities take care of and show their appreciation to the staff. I strongly encourage you to say "thank you" when deserved; as it so often goes unsaid. My partner and I used to have so many families say to us "I can't believe the change; you are great." I always replied to them, "Please send a note to the staff members; they are the ones who deserve the accolades." Often people did just that or wrote a note to the opinion page of the local newspaper. The staff beamed for days.

9. Patients'/Residents' Rights

Let me start this very important section with an example: An old farmer, who had been a hermit since the death of his wife, was found wandering aimlessly and was brought to our center. He resembled Santa Claus in coveralls, but the overpowering aroma that emanated from him could be smelled for miles. A dear, caring

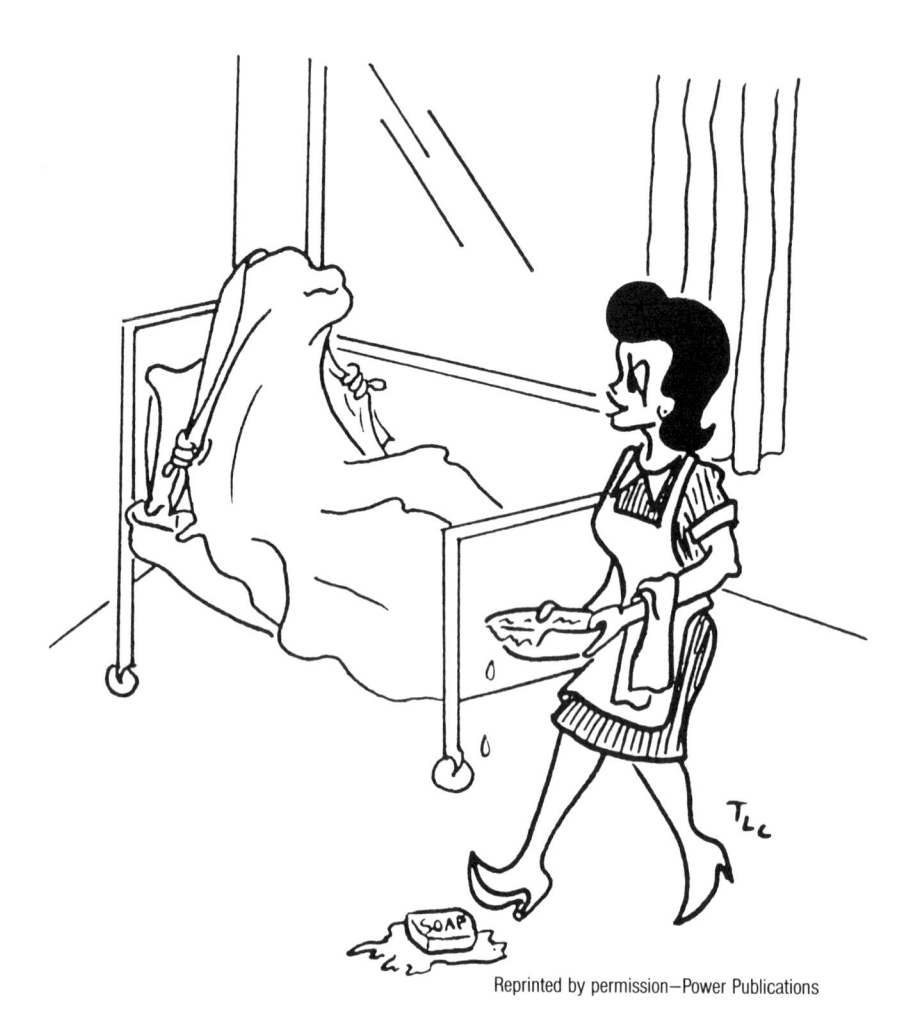

"Come on, a little soap and water never hurt anyone."

nurses' assistant went in his room and they hit it off immediately; he was obviously a ladies' man, flirting and joking with her. "I need to take you to the shower, change and wash your clothes," she said, "And then you'll feel like a new man." He raised his cane and shouted, "I ain't bathed in years, and I ain't going to start now!"

She smiled sweetly and backed out of the room and came to me for help. This is the kind of a challenge that a psychiatric nurse thrives on. I adored him, and he knew it. I told him my name and that I was a registered nurse. Thank God, he liked me! We quickly moved to a first-name basis—Homer and Lynn, old friends and old buddies. At what I thought was just the right moment, I said, "Come on Homer, it's time for a shower."

"No way," he said. Funny, my method had always worked before, I thought. So I said, "O.K. Come on, let's go to the dining room for lunch." The room was filled with women. Of course, aroma and all, he charmed them, and he was in his glory.

You guessed it—when we got back to his room, he said, "I think I'll soak in a hot tub now, but I want my same clothes." So while he soaked, we washed. He was as content as a bug in a rug from then on. He never asked to go back to his farm. Why should he? He had love, attention, and ladies—a full harem—at his beck and call.

I hope that you can see from this very classic example how residents' rights are to be respected. Yes, Homer obviously needed a bath. The nursing facilities live with a requirement that residents are to be given, or take a full bath twice a week, or as often as necessary to provide optimum care. However, had we forced the bath issue with Homer, the outcome would have been horrendous. So lots of love, skill and thought must go into the approach toward a resident. Every resident is unique and special and must always be treated accordingly. Their quirks, idiosyncrasies, routines, and preferences must always be taken into account, ditto their special customs and value systems.

Obvious problems with state and federal regulations as they relate to people are omnipresent. Blanket rules and regulations do not always take into account the human factor. So the facility is often in conflict between being in compliance with all the rules and allowing for individual freedoms of choice and preference. It is a tough balancing act, bordering on the impossible, some say.

By law each facility is required to give you a copy of the Residents' Rights Policy at the time of admission, though you may request a copy when you take a tour. In essence the rights are to assure that a resident will be guaranteed a dignified existence, and that all residents are entitled to make decisions about their care, provided each is competent to do so.

Such rights are virtually the same at all nursing homes. The importance placed on *taking the rights beyond the printed words* and the core essentials may vary greatly. The best facilities will have trained their staffs on the finer aspects of residents' rights and the importance of encouraging patients to achieve their full potential through positive attitudes. Through a combined effort (encouraged resident plus a caring, informed staff) many residents can and do improve. See Chapter Three for a synopsis of Residents' Rights.

The nursing home industry is a *service* industry, and that's exactly its reason for being—to serve people. It does not exist to serve the needs of the owners or the staff. Thus, a person should be able to go into a facility and do his or her own "thing", within reason of course. If that means staying up until 2 a.m. to watch the late show, that's exactly and precisely what the resident should be able to do in the healthcare center. If the resident is accustomed to having a beer at night, and his doctor as well as his condition permits, the resident should have that beer at night.

Watch out for certain words you may hear as you are given the tour: Expressions such as *"We don't allow"* or *"We have rules about this and that..."* If the focus is on what they do not allow, the focus is facility oriented. The focus should be on the *people principle* as in what are *your* needs, or what does your family member need to make his/her stay a more positive experience? If that means that Uncle Henry will only watch the Cubs game on TV if he can put on his bib overalls and have a beer and popcorn, then that's exactly the way it should be, and by the way, that comes within the Residents' Rights Guidelines.

10. Adult Day Care

There are many alternatives to nursing home care: Home Health Care, the Visiting Nurse Program, various state home-bound programs, Adult Day Care—all kinds of services are available. Thank God! No one should ever be in an institution—whether a hospital or nursing home or wherever—unless they need to be there for intensified care, treatment or rehabilitation, or they choose to live there and make it home. The half-step between home care and institutionalization is called Adult Daycare. It offers families a physical and mental respite from the 24-hour responsibility of caring for an elderly or dependent adult family member. It can also provide stimulation and social contact for a senior citizen who lives alone and is confined within his/her four walls. Most of the adult daycare programs will accommodate a flexible schedule, once the part-time resident has qualified for this type of care.

Initially, an interview with the prospective senior and/or family member will establish the social and medical history. A recent medical exam by a physician and the results of a current chest X-ray are a few of the requirements. The details of the social history and its importance are covered in Chapter Four. Special services are often available for the daycare resident: bathing, restrictive diets, and hair care are a few. The temporary resident is able to broaden his/her horizons through contacts with the staff and residents, and by participating in optional activities and programs.

The caregiver is able to have some measure of peace of mind during the time that the family member is at the healthcare center. Often an elderly family member must be alone during the day, sitting and looking at the four walls with only the TV for a companion. This pattern often forces passivity. Many times there is no stimulation, no joy, no involvement with people and the outside world. Your local Area Agency on Aging will be able to tell you which healthcare facilities offer adult daycare. They will also be able to tell you if there is any financial aid available for participation in this program and the requirements for obtaining it.

I know a woman who ran through the aisles of the grocery store—just throwing stuff in her cart, because she felt that she only had twenty minutes. If she didn't get back home in that short time, she feared that something terrible would happen to her husband, an Alzheimer's victim. By the time she arrived home, she couldn't remember what she bought—or why, and she was too exhausted to cook it. By bringing her husband to the Adult Daycare Program for two days a week, she received a much needed rest, and she gained some free time for herself.

My partner and I started the Adult Daycare Program at our nursing home in response to the need of a very dear man. His wife—in her 50's—suffered from two debilitating diseases. The husband was completely engulfed by the responsibility of his wife's care. In addition, the husband had to comfort and counsel a teenage daughter in the home who was devastated by her mother's illness, as well as juggle his high-level professional career at the local university. He hurried home each day during his lunch hour to feed and care for his wife. His evenings were spent preparing meals, feeding her, and only ended after bathing her, cleaning up and getting her "settled in." He was usually too exhausted to even read the paper or watch TV. His devotion to her was a full-time endeavor, and he barely recognized any of his own needs.

The Adult Day Care Program enabled this devoted man and his family to at least surmount some of the time-consuming problems that were so devastating to their individuality. When the time came that the wife needed 24-hour nursing care, the transition from part time to full time residency was easier for her and her family. The husband continued to visit every evening to nurture and reassure her "he would always be there for her." Soon, he became a regular evening volunteer, and a much needed friend to many of the other residents. I believe the nursing home experience was a positive, soul-touching one for him.

Respite (short term) care is the ideal answer to the question, "What will we do with mother/father when we go on vacation?" We spoke with relatives who had not been on vacation in five years because of the commitment of caring for a family member. Some of the prospective short-term residents will exhibit resentment initially upon being admitted, but most adapt to the new surroundings soon after the family member leaves.

We were sometimes amazed at the ability of a seemingly frail senior citizen to bamboozle his/her family members into believing that it was their absolute duty to provide constant care—no exceptions. It is chiseled in stone! When this same domineering senior citizen experienced the company of his/her peers, he/she often realized that life is a giving as well as a

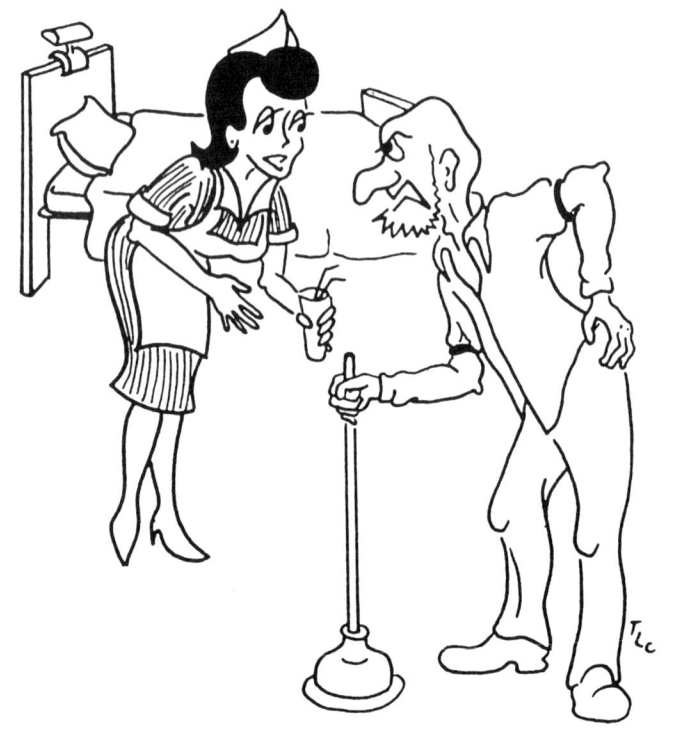

"Call my daughter and have her bring my cane."

Reprinted by permission—Power Publications

"taking" preoccupation with self. Most really do want to "give" if only asked and encouraged to do so. For many this short-term stay gave them a new perspective. Often when a person experiences the problems others face, their own seem to diminish in comparison.

Please note, that this book is about the selection of a nursing home. It does not attempt to delve into all the alternatives and choices available to you. There seems to be much written on the alternatives, but there are people for whom the nursing home choice is the decision at hand. It goes without saying that no one should ever be there unnecessarily. Most will never need to reside permanently in a nursing home, but many will be in need of rehabilitation or treatment services in those settings. I must add that many residents have told me that their quality of life was greatly enhanced in a secure, healthy, loving environment. They call it "home" and that, after all, is the mark of a good one.

11. Restoration and Rehabilitation

Together with the many other misconceptions and myths still hanging in the air, there also remains the misnomer that a nursing home is a dreaded place to go and die. Is it any surprise that people shun and fear this grim reaper scenario? In fact, the traditional emphasis on comfort care is only one facet of the services rendered in a modern healthcare center. However, for those people suffering from terminal disease, such as the terminal stage of cancer, and those who have chosen to refuse all treatment, the primary focus of rendering loving, comfort care is still appropriate. There is a separate chapter dealing with advanced directives, etc. on page 55.

Aside from the above mentioned group and the individual's right to choose, the majority of older adults can and do benefit from an individualized treatment or plan of care that emphasizes capacity versus incapacity.

First, I would define restorative care as a plan that utilizes the various disciplines (medical, therapies, nursing, dietary, activities, etc.) to restore the person to his/her optimum level of independence. This includes physical as well as emotional well-being and self-esteem. As we all know, the mind and body are so obviously co-mingled that if one feels depressed, useless, and dependent, the bodily functions will deteriorate and become dysfunctional as well.

Webster defines *restore* as: "to bring back to a former and better state; to repair, renew, and to recover." As a prospective resident or family member, you will be asked questions pertaining to A.D.L.'s. This simply means the *activities of daily living*. These may be divided into three groups described as:

1. **Self care activities.** Can the person take care of his own hygiene (bathing, teeth, toilet needs, dressing activities, including buttons and shoelaces; cooking and feeding abilities; general appearance—hair, nails, shaving)?
2. **Ambulation.** Can the person get around independently indoors and out? Can the person climb stairs? Get in and out of a car? Does the person need or use a walker, cane, or leg brace?
3. **Communication.** Can the person communicate? Express needs and problems? Comprehend verbal or written directions? Use the telephone or the help or call button?

Before the Tour 35

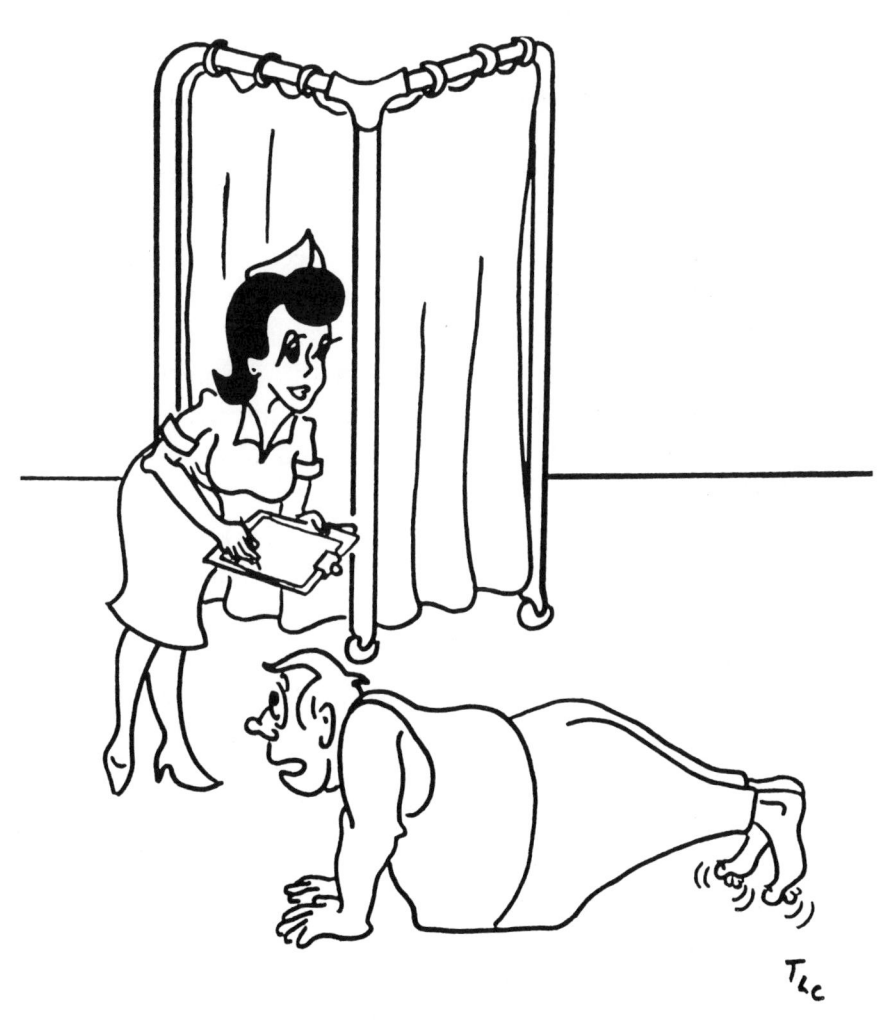

"How can I do push-ups?"

Reprinted by permission—Power Publications

Rehabilitation is defined by Webster as: "to restore to a former capacity; to re-establish in the esteem of others." In the medical world, rehabilitation generally means a team approach, involving the staff, and appropriate therapists (physical, occupational, speech, and respiratory) to evaluate and render treatment according to diagnosis, need, and responsiveness to treatment. A simple example would be the diagnosis of a fractured hip with an evaluation by a physical therapist. This therapist would work on ambulation techniques, strengthening, and this would then be carried over by the rest of the team in a collaborative effort. A major component of all rehabilitation is to focus on the strengths and abilities of the person rather than on his/her weaknesses and/or disabilities. An attitude of realistic optimism prevails, in that to achieve one must believe.

Generally, there are small gains to be made if not always a cure. These may be a series of small important steps to accomplish new coping methods and a renewed sense of goal-oriented efforts towards increased self-sufficiency. What a major triumph for a stroke victim to be able to feed oneself again! Having to be dependent and having to be fed is demoralizing and depressing. For a person who will probably not be able to return home because of numerous chronic health problems, the fact that this person is still trying helps dispel pessimism. Difficult as it is to live without hope, most older adults still believe that "hope does spring eternal." Remember an optimistic attitude enables people to achieve more and to age more comfortably with better health, according to the experts. The staff will admit that it is easier to "do for" a resident, because it takes less time. However, staff members also feel a renewed sense of achievement when they see the positive results of their efforts in enhancement and enrichment of the quality of someone's life. Let me emphasize that the rendering of restorative care is *preventative* as well. For those for whom a cure and a return home is not achievable, this type of care will help prevent contractures, incontinence, and other "lack of use" anomalies that sometimes lead to such undesirable results as people reverting to a fetal position—definitely *not* quality of life.

So as you tour and check the facility, you may easily observe the attitude and application of rehabilitation personnel and programs. Are staff people walking with residents, transferring people out of those hard, uncomfortable wheelchairs to regular "comfy" chairs? What is happening in the therapy department? Is there an on-going exercise program for all levels of participation?

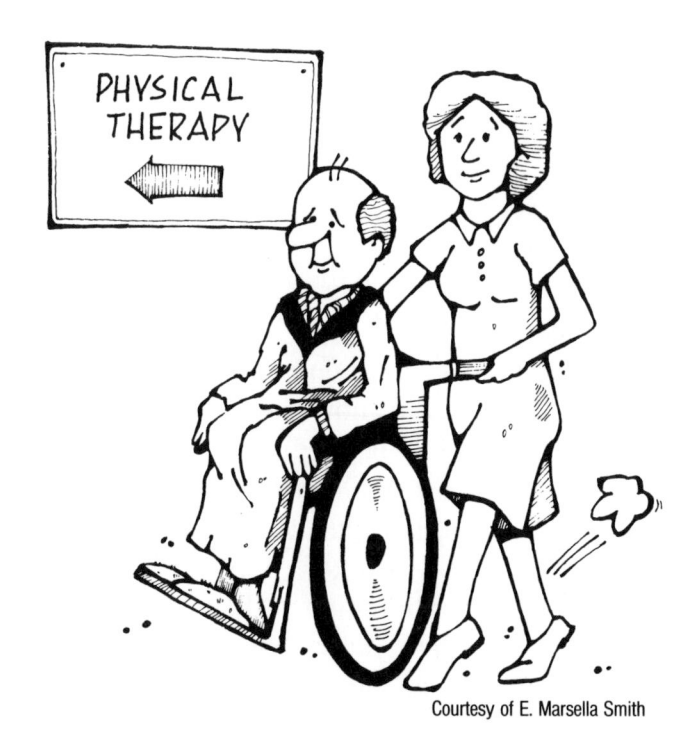

Courtesy of E. Marsella Smith

12. Observe the Resident

Look into the eyes of the residents as well as at their overall appearance. Do they appear clean and well-groomed? Are nails clean and trimmed? Are the men shaved? Remember that self-concept is directly related to how one looks and feels. Ask any woman if she doesn't "feel better" after having her hair done. Of course, she does. Residents have the same feelings and needs as you do. A resident should *never* be present in the lounge (residents' living room) in disarray, with spilled food on clothing, or clothes on backwards. In my view this is inexcusable. Are the residents dressed appropriately— appropriate to what they want to wear? Some of the women may choose to wear pant or sweat suits; some never wear slacks, but always a dress to look "proper." Observe those taking care of the people. Do they do it affectionately, kindly, with sensitivity and attention to individual needs? Is there touching? Is there genuine involvement? Do you see staff walking with residents to bolster self-esteem in regaining a higher level of functioning? How many people are in wheelchairs? Residents in wheelchairs should be properly positioned for correct body alignment, and should be wearing appropriate shoe wear. Observe people wearing glasses; are they clean and clear?

Do the residents seem content and happy? Does the center try to meet the individual's needs and wants, and make him/her feel needed? A resident may like to stay up and watch TV until midnight, or get up at 6 a.m. for coffee. Perhaps dad likes to drink a glass of wine each evening before dinner. The emphasis should always be on the continuation of these preferences, not on emphasizing rules. You can watch to see whether residents seem to be engaged in doing their "own thing."

Before the Tour 39

Just before we sold our nursing home, we had four young men in their twenties who had been involved in vehicular accidents, two of them in motorcycle accidents without helmets. It was a distressing sight, believe me. Yet these people were trying to get better and stronger with the hope of eventually going home or at least of being less dependent. So as you take your tour, and you see things that are not always pleasant, remember that the nursing home has a wide gamut of care needs. If you look beyond the obvious disfigurement and/or disability and really *see* the unique person there, you will find yourself much less bothered or offended. You may actually get involved with many residents, and find very pleasant and rewarding experiences just waiting for you to make them happen.

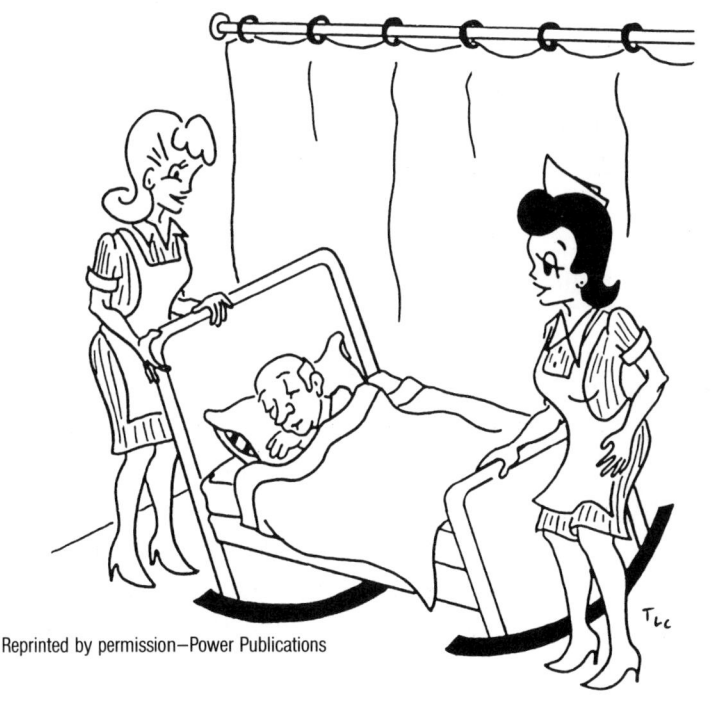

Reprinted by permission—Power Publications

"It's the only way I could get him to sleep."

13. Resident Council

At each facility, a Resident Council forms its own rules, elects officers, and functions as an independent group. Its members meet to discuss concerns and address problem areas, and to make suggestions and recommendations to various departments and to the governing body of the facility. This group is open to all residents and they meet privately without staff present. You may wish to speak to the president of the Resident Council, and to look at the minutes of its most recent meeting. Contrary to what some believe, council meetings are not just "gripe" sessions, but often a highly effective tool that helps enrich and enhance the quality of life in the facility. Let me tell you about two of many suggestions that came from our Resident Council:

1. "Let's bring snow in and build a snowman in the lobby." We *did* and it was smashing (as well as smushy) fun. The housekeeping department was great about it. They cordoned off an area, so no one would slip, and cleaned up after the Grand Masterpiece melted!

2. "How about a real live horse for all to see and touch?" That's right; we did it, brought a horse into the great room! We got wonderful responses from people who had not previously related to many of the other activities. Many residents had their pictures taken sitting in the saddle. They carried the pictures and the memories around a long time and told anyone who would listen "all about it." It was a magnificent success.

Before the Tour

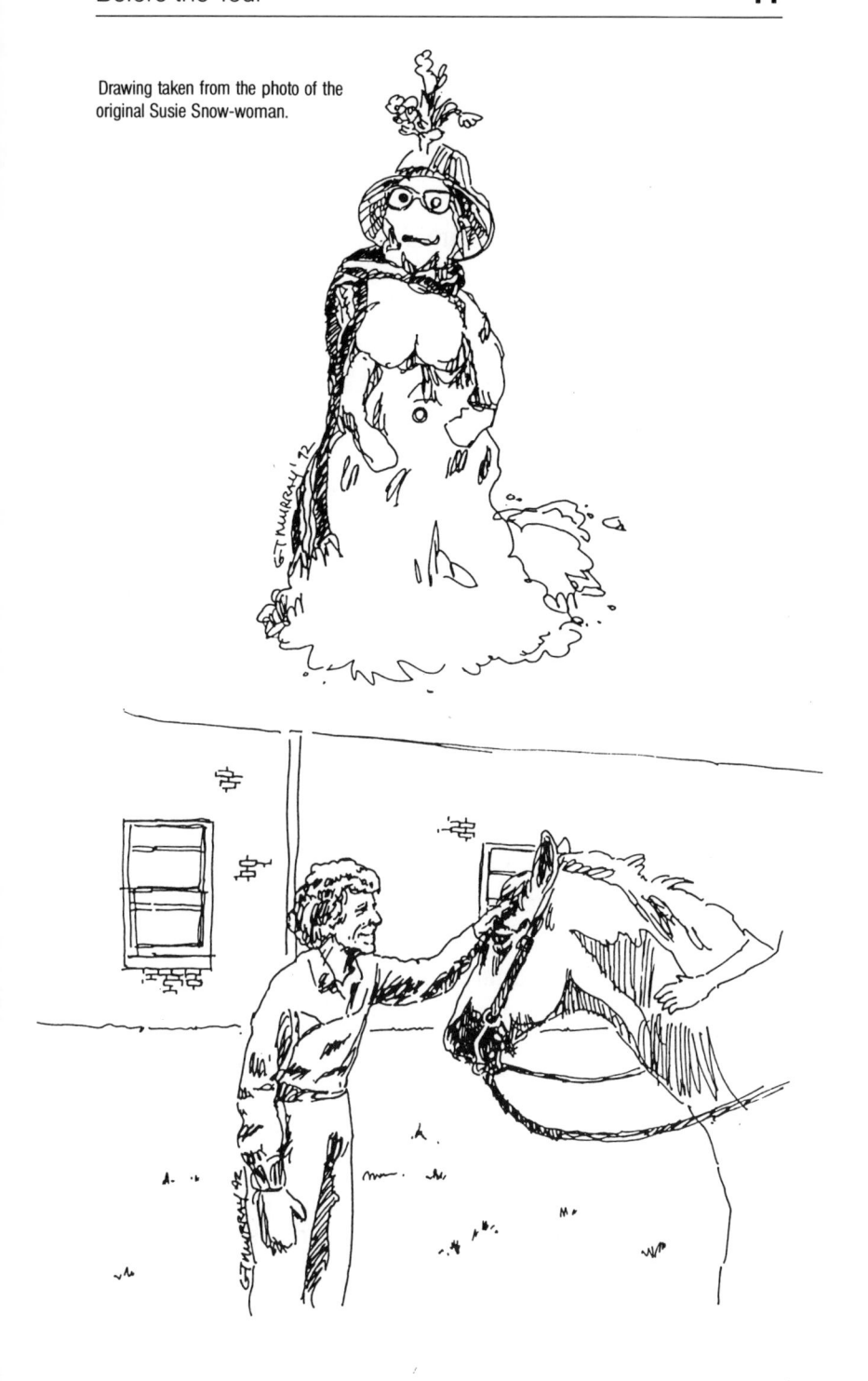

Drawing taken from the photo of the original Susie Snow-woman.

14. Dietary

Observe a mealtime if possible. The aroma and presentation should be pleasant. The weekly menu should be posted for all to see, so you should check to make sure that what is listed on the menu is actually being served. The best facilities may offer you a meal, so that you may taste and learn what the fare is like. Also go to the kitchen area and look inside. You are not permitted to be in the kitchen for reasons of sanitation. However, you can observe whether it appears sparkling, clean and organized.

But let me tell you this: a recent newspaper article about "unsanitary" conditions in the kitchen of a nursing home resulted because the state regulators cited the home for a violation for crumbs on the counter. But the reason was not explained in the article. The survey team walked into the kitchen right after the staff prepared breakfast. Now it is really tough to prepare toast for 100 or more people without getting crumbs on the counter. So we need to be fair and knowledgeable about these things. Before the new method of surveillance went into effect, many, if not most, deficiencies cited against nursing homes were paper violations. This meant some form or paper was not dated and "dotted" correctly. Now, fortunately the *emphasis* is all focused on *resident rights* and *empowerment*. This should make resident care and the outcome of the care more easily identified for you on survey reports you check. As a nurse, I am pleased because the nurses can pay more attention to people and less to paper.

Ask if substitute foods are offered in place of the daily menu. Is the food fresh, hot, and tasty? Selective menus are popular, as well as are salad and dessert carts. Many residents prefer to use a selective menu and *choose* their own entrée, vegetables, dessert, and so on. Sometimes caregivers will help the residents with their choices. Separate menus are provided for those on restrictive or therapeutic diets. The focus should always be on encouraging adults to *choose* for themselves as much as possible. If selective menus are not offered, at the very least, alternatives should be available. The best facilities have a "Kitchen Korner" for the residents where coffee, hot tea, and so on are available. Fresh fruits should be available. Some facilities offer these on a regular basis as part of the dessert cart or evening snack. Residents love the taste of fresh fruits such as cherries, peaches, apples, or strawberries. They love to choose "which one for today." Fruit is natural food and, with a proper diet and exercise, can assist in proper elimination.

A patient moved to our facility merely because her former nursing home refused to make meal substitutions. The woman who transferred could not stand fish. Every time fish was on the menu, she requested a hot dog. They wouldn't grant this simple request. A nursing home does not have the financial resources to provide short-order cooking for each individual resident. However, within reason, a resident should be able to choose a substitute or arrange through the food committee to have a special request, such as fried green tomatoes, on the menu occasionally.

One way to assess the overall dietary program is to examine the creativity of the food service plan. Any approach that de-institutionalizes food and meal times should be looked on favorably. For example, when you observe a meal, you will get a feel for whether the various dining rooms resemble a military school with bodies mechanically and obediently going through the motions only. Are people hurried along to get on to the next thing on the facility's agenda? This should be a signal that the overall philosophy of this particular facility might be schedule and rule-oriented towards the needs of the facility and not those of the residents. It's on your list of positives when you find a place that sets a tone of social, conversational meal times, evidenced by the overall ambience of the dining room, the seating, and table settings, blooming flowers in season, centerpieces, bright tablecloths and napkins.

Another key feature is the offering of "theme" dinners—cookouts (most everyone loves hamburgers, hot dogs or steaks on the grill) and social/cocktail hours. These events are scheduled on the activities calendar; ask to see it. Having an old-fashioned ice cream social is great fun for the residents and their families. Does the facility offer these kinds of special events?

A typical social hour might occur two hours prior to the evening meal. There could be a selection of a favorite cocktail, beer, wine, juice or soda, cheeses, hors d'oeuvres, and such. Lemonade or mocktails can be provided for those who choose not to drink alcohol. In the background, there could be a tape playing favorites from the 30's and 40's. On some occasions a pianist could play and take requests. The basic premise here is to reawaken social modes of behavior, to rekindle old, favorite memories.

The most important aspect of all is that these *people are treated and respected as adults* who can and do make at least some of their own choices. Because of the intrinsic make-up of a nursing home, requiring some order and scheduling, it is still imperative that the facility find creative ways to encourage residents to continue to make choices and decisions.

Before the Tour 45

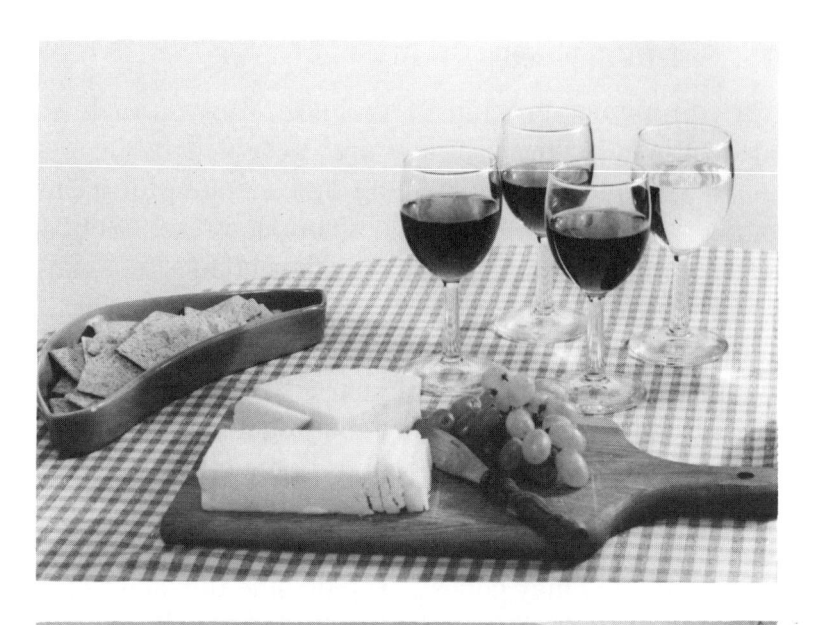

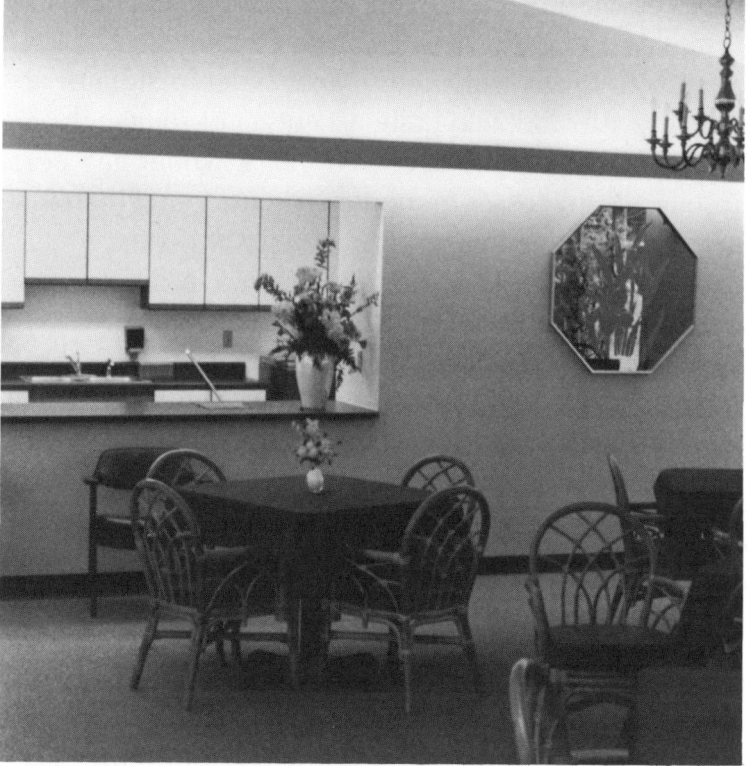

15. Spiritual Needs

Varied religious programs are almost always provided in healthcare centers. Many are presented in an ecumenical mode to be appealing and meaningful to as many as possible. Some denominations present actual services daily or weekly on a regular schedule. You may wish to contact your minister, priest, rabbi, or pastor to request continued pastoral care—something usually within the creed of most religions. Your church leader will be able to tell you of other congregational members who are at the healthcare center. Some churches send visiting committees to call on members at facilities periodically or to entertain especially at holiday times. Able residents may choose to go outside the facility for services or other church functions. Many facilities have a weekly Bible study club. Some residents ask a staff person to "pray with me." Most older residents are "tight" with God, and quite accepting of the death and dying process. This age group as a whole has been through many losses, experienced much, and therefore seems more able to accept the reality of death.

    I can also say that the staff in most facilities follow a kind of unwritten policy and philosophy in regard to the care of a dying person. It is not generally a formalized exercise, but a genuine caring process that simply evolves. It is heartwarming as the staff works out a system of making sure "someone is there" at all times. They will sit by the bedside, holding a resident's hand, talking to or praying with, simply *being there* to offer love and support. Staff members often remain at the facility on their own time to do this, simply because they really care. The idea that "one gets used to people dying" simply is not true from my experience. The staff becomes deeply involved with the residents and feels a great sense of loss when a resident dies. Tears are shed and grief is felt, as in the death of any loved one. As I said earlier, most staffers at a healthcare center are really special people.

16. Activities

The best facilities meet the residents' psychosocial, emotional and spiritual needs, as well as their medical and nursing needs. This chapter deals with the psychosocial needs as they relate to activity/recreational therapy. The calendar of activity programs will be posted. Look it over carefully. If it consists mostly of bingo and basketweaving, and your interest is in Bach and chess, there may be a problem. A therapeutic activity program will go far beyond fun and games to act as a catalyst that increases social interaction and functioning.

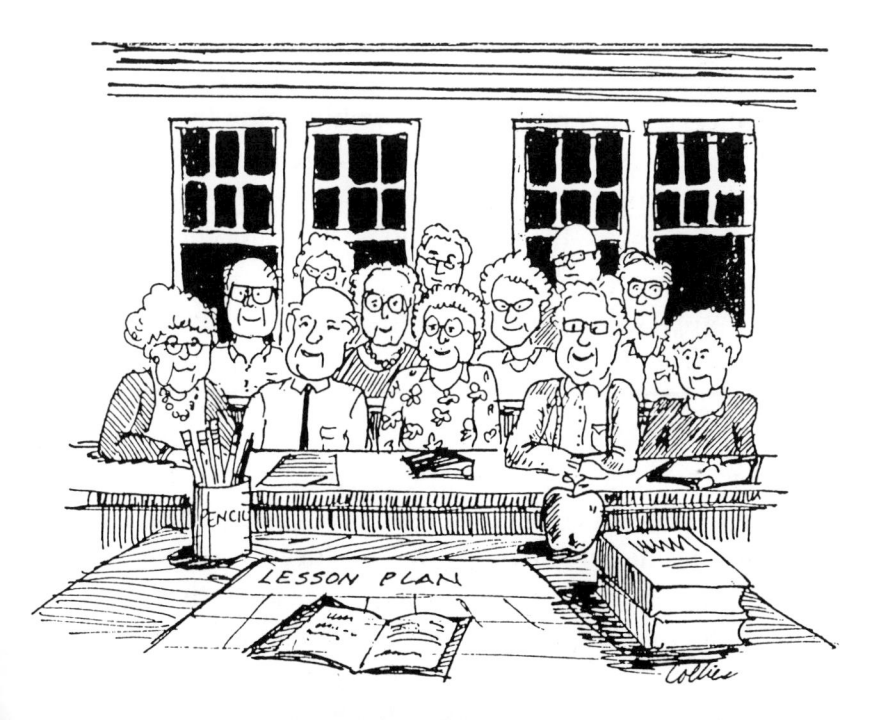

What is happening as you make your tour? Obviously the center has a wide diversification of people with a medley of interests, and the calendar should reflect that. If there is not a wide variety on the calendar, including weekend activities, ask why. No reason exists as to why any activity program can't be expanded. There are a lot of volunteers out there who love to help. Often, people from AARP and university retirees are willing to teach and present programs on a wide variety of subjects: classical music; creative writing; computers and accounting; living history, to mention only a few. Discussion of current events is a great stimulant, as are exercise and cooking classes.

While some of these programs may seem a bit ambitious for many residents, one surely enjoyed by most is the "living history." It is very gratifying to hear how eagerly many residents can recall facts from yesteryears, and how the facts that are related by one person will open a memory frame for another person. One lady at our nursing home was adept at leading an assembly of residents and often would begin by asking, for example, "Who remembers the store that was at the corner of Main and Fourth Streets in the 1940s?" A scenario of happy times evolved as pleasant memories of youth are revived and shared.

All proposed activities require a critical review; many older people object to child-like and "foolish" recreation. Some feel that certain activities are dehumanizing; a philosophy of "to each his own" should prevail. *These people are adults, not children.* Any truly effective activity program goes far beyond the monthly birthday parties and bingo games. However, for many these are quite special events so let's not put them down. A star should be given to those facilities which go far beyond

Before the Tour   49

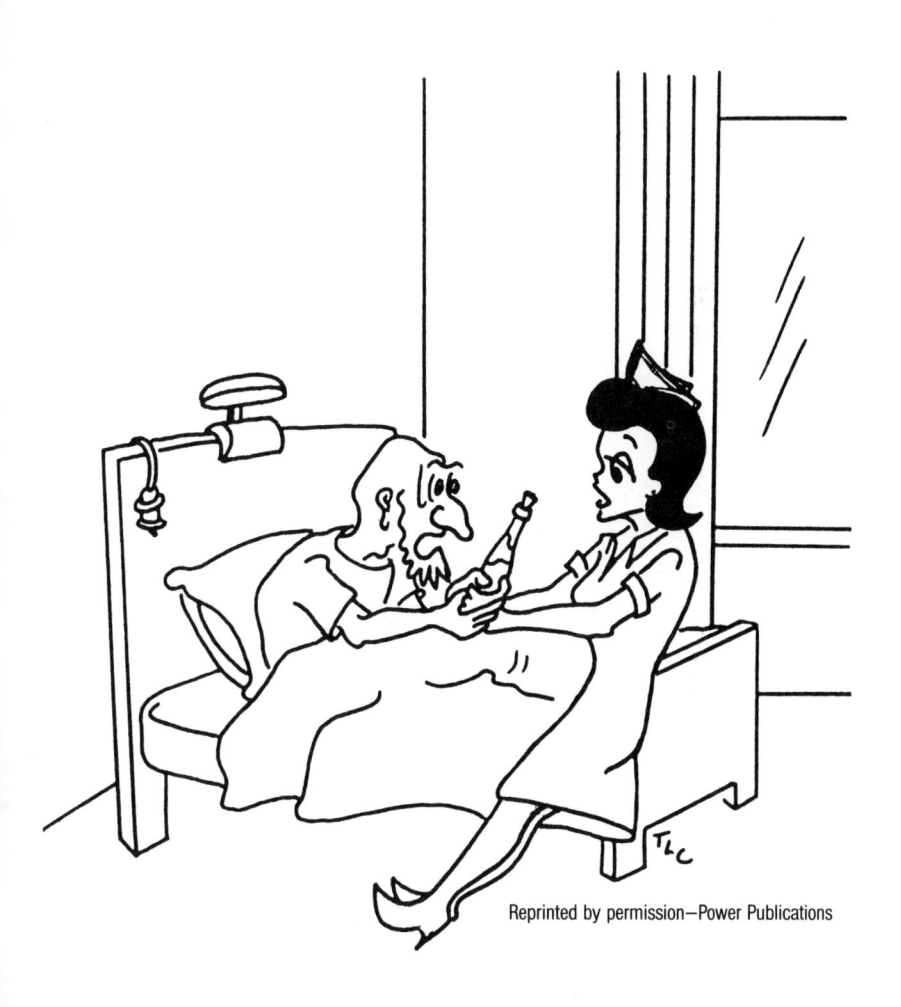

"No booze! How do you think I got to be 101?"

what is required and provide pet and music therapy, to name two.

A good signal to you regarding the activity program would be the "people-involved-with-people" principle. Do you sense a bonding process—a genuine caring about each other? Do the residents in the activity room seem lively and responsive? Does the activity calendar post a shopping trip outside the center for the residents to purchase his/her own things, as well as other trips out of the center? Does the facility have a van for these outings? Are there patio parties to get people outside? Is there popcorn, beer and basketball viewing for the guys (and the ladies like to come too)? Is there a plan to integrate the community into the planning of events? The facility shouldn't be isolated from the community; residents need to remain involved and connected to it.

As I mentioned, some people like a beer or cocktail, or a glass of wine. Again, let me reiterate; these are adults who make their own decisions and choices. It goes without saying that they would not hold wild, intoxicated parties. Obviously, a medical contraindication to alcohol would take priority, as would respect for anyone who philosophically or religiously objects to alcohol. Once again, it is *freedom of choice* and personal preference that prevails whenever possible.

Please remember that as we age, we do become more of what we are in our forties, fifties, and sixties. Thus a "loner" type personality into books, privacy, and research isn't likely to become Mr. Congeniality or the president of the resident council. Although, occasionally there are those who do "bloom" and "grow" late in life.

As you tour, listen carefully to the music you hear being played. It should be reflective of the tastes of the residents (big band sound, music of their era) and not too loud, hard rock, or rap. The new wave of music can and should be demonstrated at a music program or class, but the overall tunes emanating from the intercom should be soft.

Programs that link children of all ages (pre-school through college) are quite successful in bridging the generation gap. Ask if the facility has student affiliation programs.

Our Version of "Rapture"

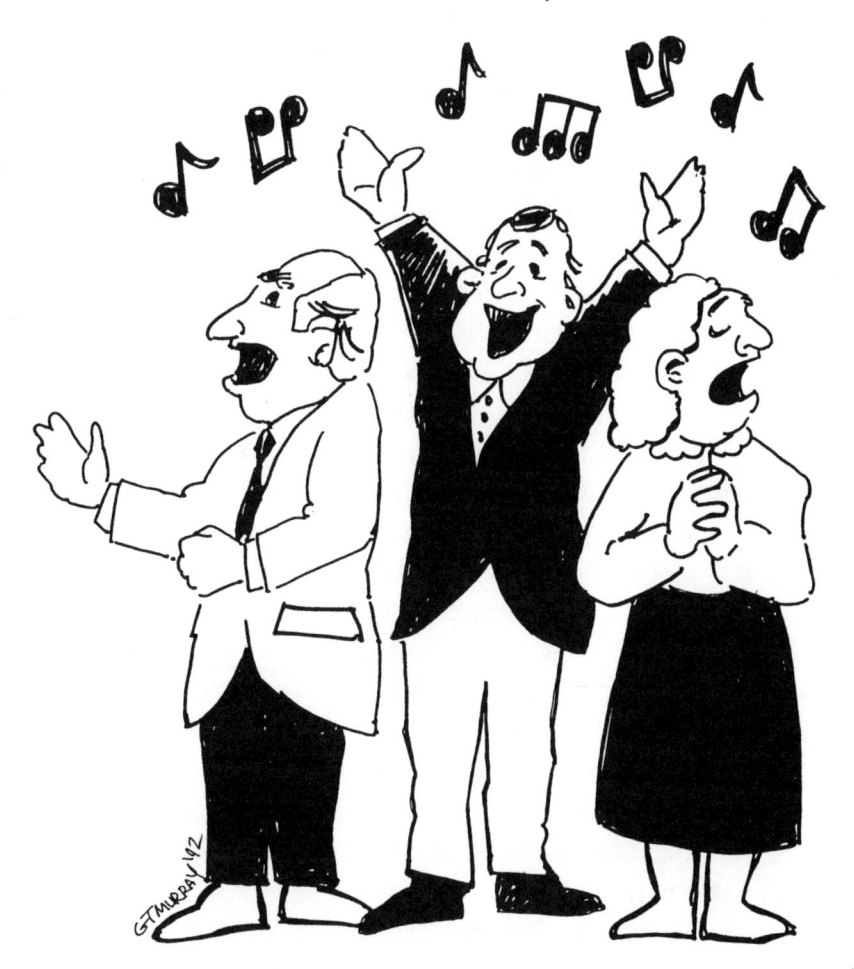

Music therapy or programs such as kitchen bands or sing-a-longs are a wonderful way to bring the joy and fun of music to everyone. For those residents with memory impairments, the rote memory of old favorite songs have people singing who can't ordinarily complete a full sentence. To hear them sing the correct verse of a song, or see them tap their feet and dance gives the resident's family and the facility staff such an indescribable high. At our facility, there were Big Band Days twice a week. The activity director, head housekeeper, a volunteer pianist and the administrator (I was the only one off key!) took to the microphone for several hours. We all took turns carrying the microphone out into the audience to encourage the residents to sing out and along. We discovered many beautiful voices and many closet "hams" who loved being center-stage performers. There was a carpenter of German descent who often waltzed with the ladies. We always sang *Amazing Grace, Rock of Ages,* and *God Bless America,* because almost everyone remembered the old spirituals and the patriotic tunes. Then we "traveled" from Vienna to New York then New York to Chicago ("that toddling town") and to special-request time after our musical journey.

Believe me, when all "those saints finished marching in," we were exhausted but euphoric. It's hard to adequately describe the excitement, fun, bonding, and, yes, rapture of those special moments. Leo Buscaglia wrote in his book *Living, Loving and Learning* that he wanted to experience rapture. We always believed we could have shown him *our version of rapture,* and he would have loved "hugging" us (his famous trademark). For all those special times and memories, I feel blessed and enriched.

With respect to activities, please remember that the

old adage of "use it or lose it" applies to mental stimulation as well as physical activity. The older person is no different in his or her needs than the rest of us. An important one is their need to be useful, needed, and appreciated as a unique individual, as well as loved, respected, and honored. A good activity program will act as a catalyst towards a more responsive involvement in participating and interacting.

So you need to look for:
- ☐ The activity calendar
- ☐ Wide diversification of programs
- ☐ Creativity
- ☐ Community involvement

17. Financial

Always ask for a list of extra costs. Find out what is included in the quoted rate, and the period of time that the rate will be in effect (many facilities raise their rates annually, others more frequently). Therefore, you will be wise to ask the facility about its pattern and percentage of increases.

Ask whether there are extra charges for different levels of care. If mother goes into the facility as an intermediate care resident and has a stroke, will she be moved to a skilled unit? At what additional cost? Is all laundry included in the daily rate? Is there an exercise program included at no additional charge? Therapies (physical, occupational, speech, inhalation, etc.) almost always cost extra. Beauty/barber charges are usually extra. There should be a schedule of rates for services rendered. What nursing supplies are included in the base rate? What nursing supplies are not included?

The issue of long-term care insurance, catastrophic healthcare financing, Medicare Parts A and B, and Medicaid are constantly being studied and revised. This book does not delve into this issue except to caution you to become informed when you visit a nursing home, and to ask such questions as, "What if my mother runs out of money? Will she have to leave the facility? Do you participate in Medicaid? What are the requirements for participating in Medicaid?" If there is the possibility that Medicaid will be an option, it would be wise to also check in with your local welfare department if only to be doubly sure of eligibility conditions. Most states also have a pre-screening process to assure appropriate placement or alternative services. You may check with the Area Agency on Aging in your community as well as with your physician and social workers from your local hospitals. There is a comprehensive list of agencies listed on page 100 for further information.

CHAPTER 3

Resident Rights
Advanced Directives

Contained in the Omnibus Budget Reconciliation Act (OBRA) of 1990 is a federal law called the "Patient Self-Determination Act." The essence of it is that people can express their wishes regarding treatment in the form of "advanced directives." An advanced directive is the general term for a written statement that is prepared in advance of a serious illness. The use of an advanced directive is a way to control your future medical treatment. It could be a living will or durable power of attorney for health care. This assures compliance with your decisions before a situation arises where you can no longer make a health care decision for yourself.

Please consult your lawyer for expert legal opinion and advice. This chapter deals only with the major aspects of the law, and not your particular needs and requests. Noteworthy is the fact that each state will have particular regulations and laws that may vary, so you must check the laws in your state.

The new federal law requires providers in the federally funded Medicare and Medicaid programs to *inform* adult patients about their *rights* to *refuse* or *accept medical treatment.* This requirement to inform must be documented in the records of an adult person in a hospital, nursing home, hospice, health maintenance organization (HMO), or under home healthcare programs. You are *not* required to have an advanced directive—only to be advised of your right to execute one should you wish. Put simply, advanced directives can protect your right to decide in advance of an extreme medical condition such as permanent coma, terminal illness, or irreversible brain damage.

A living will may not be recognized in all states—or there may be special, legal forms and documents required by each state. A living will expresses your wishes regarding life-support systems, should you have a terminal condition. Treatment choices can be included or excluded. Some of these life-prolonging measures are intravenous therapy (IV's), respirators (a ventilator machine), feeding tubes and CPR (cardiopulmonary resuscitation).

A durable power of attorney for health care is a written document in which you designate a person to act as your agent or proxy who is authorized to make healthcare decisions for you which you are unable to make for yourself (by reason of incompetence or unconsciousness). Each provider (in this case, the nursing home) must have written policies regarding all aspects of resident rights, including policies on advanced directives. The facility has the obligation to inform you of these rights, inquire as to your wishes, educate you of your informed consent rights, and then document all this in your medical record. To clarify: "Informed Consent" means you must give your permission for care or treatment after being fully and clearly informed by your physician of the risks and gains in any procedure, surgery, or treatment planned.

Residents' Rights (Specifics)
Let me briefly explain *some* of the provisions stated in the Residents' Rights. I hope your realization that these rights are guaranteed by law will help dispel some of the mistrusts and misconceptions about nursing homes. All of the residents' rights evolved through the joint efforts of federal and state agencies, advocacy groups (American Association of Retired Persons, Congress of Senior Citizens, other senior advocacy groups, and the American Healthcare Association among others). The burden of ensuring that these rights are protected and promoted rests with the facility. Reaping as much benefit as possible from these rights is the privilege of each resident.

Each resident has the right to a dignified existence, self-determination, and communication with and access to persons and services inside and outside the facility. The resident has the right to exercise his or her rights as a resident of the facility and as a citizen or resident of the United States. The resident has the right to be free of interference, coercion, discrimination, and reprisal from the facility in exercising his or her rights. The facility must inform the resident both orally and in writing in a language that the resident understands of his or her legal rights and all the rules and regulations governing resident conduct and responsibilities during the stay in the facility.

A resident has the right to accept or refuse treatment and must be informed of the medical consequences of any refusal. His/her total health and medical condition must be explained in understandable terms, and the resident's medical records (and any other records) must be made available to him/her within twenty-four hours if requested. After receipt of his/her records, copies may be purchased at local rates if requested and given to the resident within two working days. His/her choice of a physician is guaranteed, and information about the physician (name, specialty, and method of contact) must be provided. Confidentiality of personal and medical records is absolute. Privacy must be observed in accommodations, but the facility is not required to provide a private room for each resident. Staff members should knock before entering a room, and use privacy curtains when needed. Every resident has the right to reasonable and regular access to a telephone, and any telephone or written contacts, as well as any visits, may be private if desired. Immediate access and visitation rights must be granted to the resident's physician, any representative or agency responsible for the advocacy of the resident, including the developmentally disabled and mentally ill individuals. Such rights must also be granted to immediate family members or other relatives, subject to the resident's right to deny or withdraw consent or to any others who are visiting with the resident's consent. All, of course, are subject to reasonable restrictions. Providers of health, social, legal or other services may also visit, again with the resident's right of denial or withdrawal of consent.

Each resident may retain and use personal possessions. This may include personal furnishings and suitable clothing as space, safety and health requirements allow. When married residents live in the same facility, and where both spouses agree and the arrangement is not contraindicated by the physician, they may share the same room.

Residents' Rights and Advanced Directives

The current daily rate charged by the facility must be provided to all except Medicaid patients. Written notice of any items that are not included in the daily rate, and the charges for those items and services must be provided. Medicaid patients should be given a list of charges that are not covered by Medicaid. Residents and applicants for admission must be furnished with the necessary information regarding Medicare and Medicaid benefits and eligibility. If applicable a written description of the equitable share of the spouse's community resources that can be retained while receiving Medicaid, and the spend-down provisions which may be necessary to qualify must be provided.

If a resident chooses to keep personal funds at the facility, the resident must receive a quarterly statement that accounts for those funds. If a resident has an account that exceeds fifty dollars, the facility then must keep the excess in an interest bearing account. All resident personal money must be kept entirely separate from the facility's money. In pooled accounts, there must be a separate accounting of each resident's share.

Residents have the right to complain about any condition that causes them concern. These complaints may be made to staff members, family members, the resident council, advocacy groups or individuals. The nursing home must post the names and phone numbers of the state advocacy groups and individuals, such as: the state licensure office, the local and state ombudsman program, the protection and advocacy network, the Medicaid fraud control unit, and the state survey and certification agency. These must be posted prominently, and access to a telephone and privacy to call must be provided. Any suggestion or complaint that a resident has can be made without fear of reprisal or discrimination. These grievances include any treatment or neglect or lack of treatment. This provision should be explained to the resident. *If you as a current resident or family member find yourself or your loved one in an unacceptable situation that jeopardizes safety and health, you have the right to be relocated at another facility. You may call your local Area on Aging, Nursing Home Ombudsman, or the state governing agency for immediate assistance.* These phone numbers are posted at the nursing home.

The resident may refuse to perform any service for the facility, for example the performance of work or a task. If the resident desires to do something helpful and it is documented specifically in the plan of care, it must be designated either voluntary or paid. This paid arrangement rarely occurs, but many residents love to do volunteer work at the reception desk and the like.

Changes in a resident's condition will be made known immediately to the resident. If previously designated, the resident's legal representative or family member will be notified when any of the following situations occur:

1. an accident involving the resident which results in injury and has the potential for requiring physician intervention;

2. a significant change in the resident's physical, mental, or psychosocial status (i.e. a deterioration in health, mental, or psychosocial status in either life-threatening conditions or clinical complications);

3. a need to alter treatment significantly (i.e. a need to discontinue an existing form of treatment due to adverse consequences, or to commence a new form of treatment); or the necessity of transferring or discharging the resident.

Residents' Rights and Advanced Directives

If a resident chooses to remain in a nursing home, he may do so unless one of the following conditions is present:

1. A transfer is necessary for the resident's welfare, and his/her needs cannot be met in the facility.
2. The resident's health has improved to the extent that he/she no longer needs the services provided by the facility.
3. The safety and/or the health of the individuals in the facility would otherwise be endangered.
4. The resident has failed, after reasonable and appropriate notice, to pay for (or to have paid under Medicare or Medicaid) a stay at the facility.
5. The facility has ceased to operate.

The facility must demonstrate that at least one of the above situations exists before the resident is transferred or discharged against his will.

Before a facility transfers or discharges a resident, the facility must notify the resident and, if known, a family member or legal represenative of the resident about the transfer or discharge, and the reason for the move in writing in a language and manner they would understand. This notice must be given at least thirty days in advance *unless* the safety, welfare or health of the resident would be endangered. If the resident's health has improved and no longer needs the services provided or the resident has been in the facility for less than thirty days, this notice may be made as soon as practicable (feasible) before transfer or discharge. This written notice must include the reason, the date of transfer or discharge and the location to which the resident is to be transferred. Also included would be a statement that the resident and/or legal representative

Courtesy of Reneé Smith

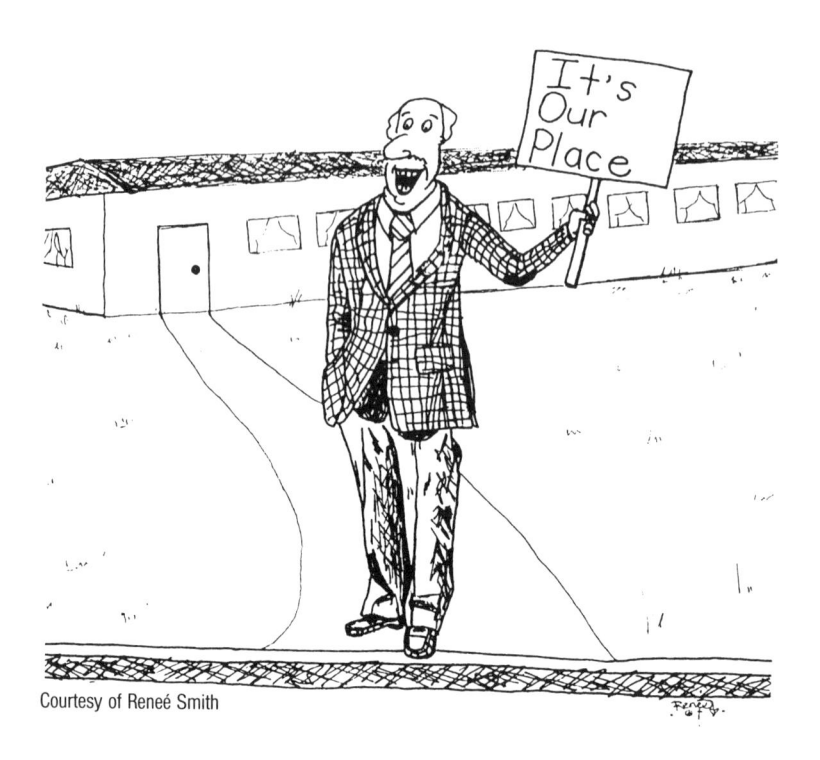

has the right to appeal this action to the state or agencies responsible for the protection of the advocacy of a particular resident.

The resident and family member will also be notified when there will be a change in the resident's room or roommate, and any change is made in the residents' rights (as mandated by federal and state regulations). The resident has the right to refuse being transferred to another room if the purpose is merely to relocate. This refusal does not affect the resident's eligibility or entitlement to Medicaid benefits. The name, address, and phone number of the resident's representative and/or family member must be recorded and updated upon notification of any change. Self-administration of drugs is allowed if the interdisciplinary team has determined that this practice is safe for a specific resident.

Residents' Rights and Advanced Directives

The results of the most recent survey of the facility, made either by federal or state inspectors, as well as any plan of correction must be available for examination upon request. The plan of correction spells out exactly how and when any omissions or unacceptable conditions will be rectified.

Each resident has the right to receive his/her own mail within twenty-four hours during the weekdays, and the mail must be unopened. The facility may only open a resident's mail when written authorization has been received from either the resident or his/her legal representative. Postage, writing paper, pens, and pencils must be available for purchase by the residents. As an amenity, some nursing homes have expanded their supply of postage stamps and writing materials to include greeting cards for special occasions and holidays. Some have a gift shop on site.

The rights discussed in the preceding are taken from the *1992 Federal Register* and are representative provisions and not all-inclusive.

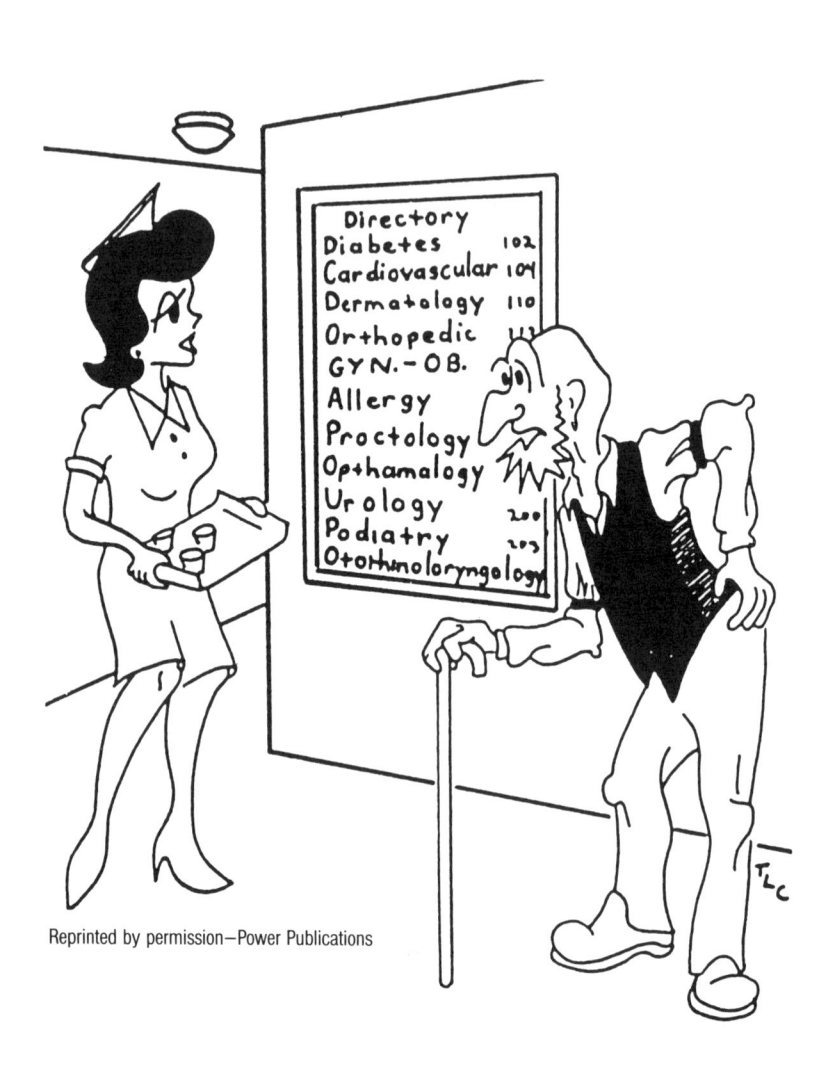

"What about the man who has everything?"

CHAPTER 4

Social History

Any professional facility will be most anxious to compile an extensive social history. The social history is a reflection of a person's past, present, and an estimate of the future. Think of all the things that have happened in a life time. Think in terms of sixty, seventy, eighty, or ninety years' worth. Do we not learn from everything we experience? We can benefit and grow—this is mental health. The more complete the social history, the better the resident can be understood, cared for, and encouraged. I hope the resident or family will be able to provide the nursing facility with the pertinent information about the resident's life, and especially all the special "little things" that are so important. What was the childhood like? Did he grow up in the home of loving parents—or was it a dysfunctional family with many unresolved hurts (abusive, alcoholics, for example)? Early in life a person may have perceived the world and the people in his life as kind, helpful, and loving, or abusive, hostile and emotionally distant. She may have been the youngest child and "babied"—or the oldest and had to "grow up" before her years. He may have been laughed at, ridiculed, or praised and held in high esteem. He may have seen himself as a winner or a loser. He may have respected authority or rebeled against it. In the work world, perhaps he was a workaholic and excelled. He may have lost jobs and fought off bill collectors. Maybe he was thought of as an asset, a success—or merely as a number. Before he married, maybe he was a "super jock" worshipped by all, or maybe a "nerd" at whom girls laughed. Maybe he still has a wife, or maybe she's dead. Maybe she walked out on him when the bill collectors came. Maybe she ran off with another man (might make him suspicious, to say the least). Rather than prying, the social history interview should provide valuable clues as to this unique, special person. Health: maybe he has always been sickly, or healthy as a horse. How does he see himself and illness? Does illness make him feel weak and unmanly? He may have been in the war and close to death, or perhaps never been sick a day in his life. This has a lot to do with how frightened a person may be. He may see the nursing home as a helping place—or as the end. He may be entering because of his family—or he may be confused. He may be waiting to live again—or to die. He may have family members who will come and visit—or he may be completely alone. Think of it, he has *no one*. Once again, this is where the caring staff steps in to become like family and dear friends.

 If the resident is unable to reconstruct the family history for the interview, the information should be obtained from the family, friends, and/or the case worker. If he has a family, they may be standing by to help when he leaves—or his family may be hoping to keep Grandpa "put away." All of these things are important in getting to know the resident as a *person*. For then, and only then, can the staff effectively communicate and understand. For example, some women prefer to be called by their first names. Others cling tenaciously to their surnames and the courtesy title, Mrs. Perhaps the woman's husband died recently, and she does not wish to relinquish the Mrs. title. Or maybe it is merely a continuation of a practice of courtesy and respect that was prevalent during her youth (to address older people by their title and last name) that she wishes to see continued. Some have nicknames, but do not want new acquaintances to use them. So, the seemingly insignificant question, "What does your mother like to be called and by whom?" really requires a thoughtful answer. Of course, the staff would ask the resident, "What would you like us to call you?" It is rarely appropriate or respectful to hear adults being called the "cutesy" names by staff. I refer to "honey," "granny," "gramps," "hun-bun," etc.

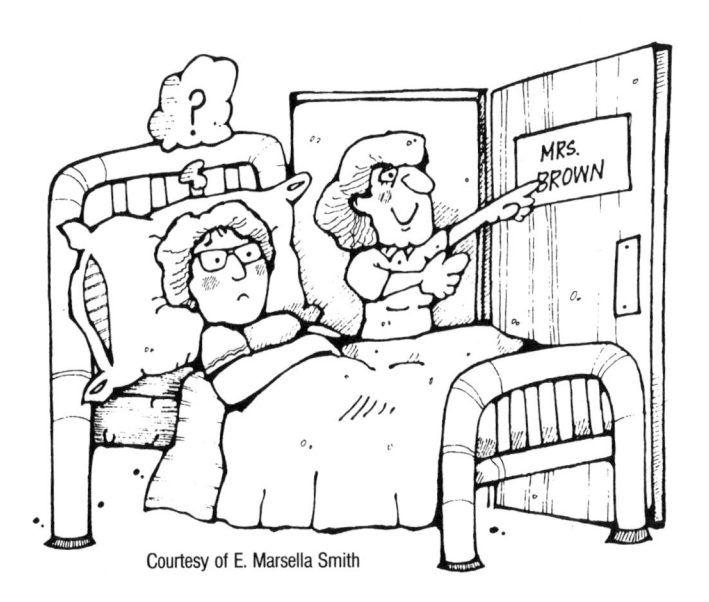

Courtesy of E. Marsella Smith

So as you tour you can listen and observe those things and assess the facility's approach to residents as people. A nice touch would be to see the resident's name on a nameplate over the resident's room, because this signifies a personalized "welcome to my place" environment.

One of our volunteers compiled an extensive background history/memoires of each resident and had them typed in a booklet form that the resident could put on the door or over the bed, etc. Sometimes it was a collage of a baby picture on through the passages and milestones of this particular life up to the present. It was a unique and neat way to open windows of conversation, particularly for those with some degree of mental impairment or memory loss. As one said, "See... I am *somebody* too."

CHAPTER 5

Psychotropic Medications & Restraints
Senility

Included in the federal guidelines, under the provision of OBRA (the Omnibus Budget Reconciliation Act), are all of the detailed regulations concerning the use of medications in nursing homes. There are some psychoactive medications (such as Thorazine, Mellaril, Haldol, to name a few) that are referred to as chemical restraints. If the action of the medication is restrictive in terms of mood alteration and behavior, then this type of medicine is considered a restraint. There are some residents, who by virtue of diagnosis and treatment, require this type of medication (schizophrenia, acute psychosis, and similar conditions), otherwise they would most probably suffer frightful distress and regression. The intent of all of these regulations is to insure proper medication therapy specific to the needs of the individual resident. A medication must *never* be given to *a resident for the purpose of staff convenience or punishment.* Simply put—never to keep a resident *"quiet"* or to *discipline* an aggressive behavior with a drug.

All medications must be monitored for appropriateness as to need and dosage, timeliness, potential drug interactions, and side effects at least once a month by a registered pharmacist. In addition, all medications are prescribed *only* by a physician and administered *only* by a licensed person. The facility must also ensure that the resident is *not* on *any* unnecessary drugs and monitor any medication errors.

Ask the tour director about the facility's policy and philosophy about medications—less is normally always better. Medications can have side effects and adverse interactions, the most common being confusion. Pills are not the instant cure for everything. Maybe the first thing we need to do is to get a medication need analysis, then try to get the resident off that "sack full of medicine" with which he came in. And most of them do come in with sacksful. No, I'm not kidding you, sometimes it has been "mix and match" medicines. We have all kinds of drugs out there that people are taking too much of—especially older people. Also, the dosage for an older person should generally be one-half the strength of what would be considered a usual adult dosage. One reason is that older people assimilate drugs faster. It is heartening to note that the pharmaceutical firms are beginning to offer medications in reduced dosage for the elderly. You may want to check this out if it applies to you or to a loved one.

In this age of specialization, we often go to one doctor for a hangnail, and another when our foot hurts. God forbid, sometimes we have seven doctors working for us. The right and left hands have no idea what medications are being taken, and the result is often a lot of drug interactions that cause depression, confusion, anxiety and a host of other symptoms. Then sprinkle in "borrowing" Aunt Tillie's arthritic medicine ("it helped her") and Uncle Harry's gout medicine, as well as two

Psychotropic Medications and Restraints—Senility

or three over-the-counter medicines and you spell disaster—not relief.

Please don't bring on trouble by using someone else's medications. A note of irony is that the symptoms that can be caused by "mix and match" medicines may then place the person in a "label-it-and-prescribe-yet-*another*-medication-to-fix-it" mode.

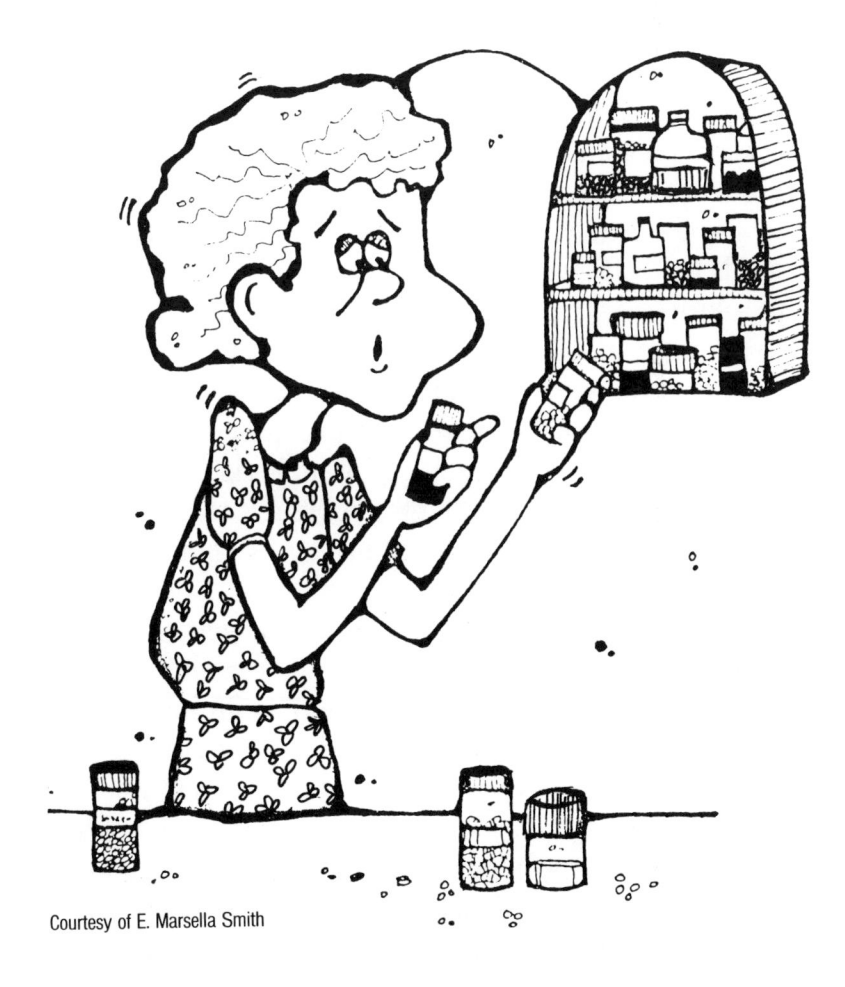

Courtesy of E. Marsella Smith

At our nursing center many times we would get credit for performing miracles, and all we had done was to take away someone's sack of medicine and get someone off all of that stuff. Imagine—taking ten pills at once. What are they all doing down there? They are probably going to interact with one another, and many times they are going to *create* increased problems rather than cure. Then, suddenly the domino theory takes effect: "Poor ol' soul, he's confused, he hasn't dressed in days; we haven't seen him, so we're going to call someone, and we're going to send him to the nursing home." Probably, he needs good and adequate nutrition as well. Most of the time, older people on low, fixed incomes who live alone do not eat well. They tend to skip around, "piece around," and fool around with good nutrition.

By the way, the term "senility" has no real meaning, nor is it an official diagnosis as such. It is only reflective of a series of symptoms. These symptoms can be related to lots of *treatable conditions.* Too often an older person is referred to as being senile merely because he or she can't remember something. "The problem with us," says Dr. Robert Butler, a leading gerontologist, "as we get older is not that we forget; the problem is that we get so darn smart that our minds are so overloaded with information that we can't store it all."

Dr. Butler concludes that only five percent of the older population actually suffer from a true organic brain syndrome that would manifest itself as an impairment of intellectual function, memory, and judgment. The experts from the National Institute on Aging and the U.N. World Assembly assert that some of the causes of these symptoms—incorrectly *labeled* senility—are surprising. Perhaps as many as twenty to twenty-five percent can be related to drugs. We are not talking about street "undercover" drugs, but about regular prescription medications properly prescribed by a physician or several physicians.

Another fifteen to twenty percent of the symptoms of senility can be caused by depression. Very often people who are depressed do not eat much at all. When you consider the mega losses (usually experienced in quiet acceptance) by this older age group, no small wonder that depression can easily set in. Left untreated, depression can lead to a negative attitude and a sense of profound helplessness. A kind of depression which can cause a sense of disorientation and confusion often follows the loss of a spouse. The person may hide away in his/her house or apartment, and may be at risk for all of the symptoms of "cabin fever." That's where life revolves around a set of four walls with virtually no stimulation or awareness of time or purpose. There follows a general fatigue, loss of interest in dressing and eating, and a general withdrawal from life. This kind of sensory deprivation itself can be responsible for another ten percent of the symptoms masking as senility. Statistics show that senile type symptoms are six times greater in people who are alone; the death rate also accelerates in lonely, depressed individuals. Obviously, the preventative key is to maintain and nurture friendships, stay active, interested, and involved.

Many nursing homes have "drug-free holidays" to encourage physicians to re-evaluate their residents' medication regimen, and to help them to see their world without all the medicines "blinding" their ability to do so. Medicines are monitored very closely in the nursing home. No drug is administered without a doctor's prescription, and the doctor has the final decision regarding any complaint of "too much." Frequently the resident is able to be weaned from the sackful philosophy of "more is better" down to the essentials only.

You may want to write for a copy of *Medicines and You: A Guide for Older Americans.* This is offered by the Council on Family Health, 225 Park Avenue S., Suite 1700, New York, N.Y. 10003.

Restraints—Physical
You may have heard that people are all "tied up and drugged in nursing homes." It is one of the most negative of all impressions of the industry. So I'll try to give you some lay terminology, knowledge, and understanding of this area of concern. Indeed, if you have visited relatives in any nursing facility, you have probably seen a resident in a wheelchair or geri-chair with a cloth restraint around the waist to keep the person from toppling over. You may have seen more than one type of restraint, or have read about the "horror" incidents.

First, let's define a physical restraint as any device that restricts freedom of movement. This would include any soft material, device or equipment which is attached or adjacent to the resident's body which cannot be easily removed by the resident. Some examples would be cloth or nylon belt or vest restraints, arm or leg restraints, hand mitts, wheelchair safety bars, as well as the geriatric type chair that has a tray that fits close to the body.

The use of, or need for, these types of restraints evolved over the primary issue of resident safety. A classic example would be a resident who is confused and unable to comprehend directions. This same resident may have had a fractured hip from a fall, and is now non-weight bearing while the area heals. However, this resident continues to try and get up and walk, and falls repeatedly, causing further injury to herself. Generally, most family members are frightened and concerned so they err on the side of safety by asking or insisting that the person be restrained to prevent further damage. The medical and nursing staff are ambivalent as well, as they feel responsible for the safety of the resident. Another example would be a person who is a "wanderer" who often attempts to leave the building to go home and "take care of the babies" (or whatever). This is a different but complex safety issue as well. Because of the many advances in technology, there are now several electronic, monitoring systems available that beep if a resident goes outside, as well as door alarms on exit doors to alert staff.

All of these electronic security devices are welcomed by the industry, because balancing freedom of movement with security and safety is an enormous dilemma for the staff. Perhaps I have been privileged with my experiences but I have always seen a reluctance on the part of the staff to use a restraint.

As a matter of fact, there has been a decided movement from within the industry itself to reduce or even eliminate restraints with considerable success. Thoughtfully cognizant of the safety issue, most of the staff know from first-hand clinical experience that restraints can aggravate the resident's physical and emotional disabilities. Most believe *dignity* and *freedom* should take first priority. Please remember, the staff is often caught in a cross fire between regulations, policies and the people principle. Generally, good old-fashioned, common sense prevails, because the more educated and enlightened staff want what's best for the resident.

Some of the less restrictive measures include pillows,

wedge cushions, pads, and a velcro safety belt; these can and should be used first if a restraint is deemed necessary. These less restrictive measures, in conjunction with a sensitivity on the part of the staff towards intervention and behavior modification, will reduce the need for restraints. The best facilities will have a restraint reduction program underway, and will be responsive to innovations and alternatives to physical restraints.

Another problem concerns the resident who may pull out an I.V. (intravenous) or N.G. (naso-gastric) tube when the resident and/or legal, durable power of attorney want all life-sustaining methods, especially nutrition, to be maintained. How many times can a resident pull out an intravenous tube, and have to have it reinserted? How much pain should be inflicted, because this resident is cognitively impaired and unaware why the tube is in place? If this is a life-threatening situation and the procedure is required for treatment (or the resident has a living will specifying, "I want this to be done"), then a restraint might well be indicated for this period of treatment.

What may have happened in the past may have been a staff mentality that said, "Well, she's always had a restraint on." "Why?" you may ask. If "I'm not sure" is the response, then this is a concern for you as you tour and ask questions. You will very easily pick up on the overall philosophy and attitude of the facility regarding their restraint policy.

CHAPTER 6

Positive Treatment Program

Perhaps you have noticed how Sophia on the TV program "Golden Girls" says, "Picture this!" Well, picture this: There's going to be a day in the very near future when persons like yourself are going to say, "Please take me to the nursing center." Here is my reason for believing this. First, under the hospital DRG program (Diagnostic Related Groupings), you are allowed a predetermined number of days to get well, based on your diagnosis and your specific illness or operation. It doesn't matter what's wrong with you in addition to the primary problem. The new system says for example, that if you've had a stroke you get seven days to get better and get out of the hospital. That may be totally wrong, but that seems to be how the system functions now.

So healthcare centers have had to become more intensive rehabilitation centers. They are stepping stones between the hospital and a return home. Many centers, if not most, were light-years ahead and have been providing this kind of treatment for many years. Unfortunately, far too many people still believe that if you go to a nursing home the door slams behind you, and you'll never get out and see the bright sunshine again. That need not be the case at all.

The U.S. Census Bureau conducted a survey in 1986 and found that 90.8 percent of the residents in healthcare facilities liked their accommodations; 91.8 percent liked the staff; 84 percent liked the relationship with other residents, and 87.3 percent liked the treatment they received. Such positive, encouraging news received limited, isolated media coverage. I envision the day when the nursing home will be the preferred treatment of choice. The operative word here is *treatment.* Most healthcare centers (sounds better than *the home*, doesn't it?) are quite knowledgeable about rehabilitation, and many are choosing to specialize in skilled care to restore people to their maximum potential. Please refer to the chapter on rehabilitation for specifics. Believe it or not, many nursing home patients do receive skilled rehabilitation, and restorative care, and are able to return home. Most people with a fracture can benefit from physical therapy. It goes without saying that rehabilitation should be an integral part of a high quality treatment program. Please remember that a fractured hip is but one segment of the whole. The emotional trauma and mind games that beset older adults are of gargantuan proportion. "I'll be an invalid," "I'm no good to anyone anymore," "I'm a burden," "I'll never walk again," These are all typical reactions. My own mother was concerned about dancing again. The worst reaction is always the theme: "Who needs me, now that I'm less than I was before, and who cares and will accept me as I am now?"

Dr. Barry Rovner, a psychiatrist at Johns Hopkins University, conducted a study of 454 residents in eight nursing homes. His findings were reported in *The Journal of the American Medical Association* where Dr.

Rovner and his associates concluded that 12.6 percent of the residents studied were severely depressed, and another 18.1 percent showed signs of depression. Their research also revealed that depressed patients had a 59 percent greater chance of dying within a year than non-depressed patients. At any given time an estimated 1.5 million people occupy American nursing homes, as many as 450,000 of those suffer from clinical depression, according to Dr. Rovner's study.

Here are some of the common symptoms of depression: a change in sleep pattern, such as awakening very early in the morning and being unable to go back to sleep; a weight loss of five to twenty pounds, accompanied by a complaint of loss of appetite. The list of physical complaints voiced by a depressed patient is seemingly endless, and may involve any organ system: constipation, headache or dizziness, pervasive fatigue, etc. If a patient complains, "I'm so depressed," it must be evaluated, certainly a medicine review would be in order. Please refer to the chapter on medications.

The best nursing centers do in fact provide excellent rehabilitation programs. If you are a resident, or a relative of a resident, insist upon such programs. If you are not getting these services, and it is within your reasonable goal to improve, get out of there and get to a facility that does provide rehabilitative services. Approximately 40 percent of all patients at our nursing center returned home within six months, so rehabilitation is a part of treatment if prescribed and desired. But regardless of what the diagnosis is, there should be a treatment program. Remember, it doesn't matter what the diagnosis is, because many of them are simply labels. Chronic brain syndrome, senility, and Alzheimer's disease have become catch-all diagnoses in some cases for the symptom of confusion. Let's make sure that a correct diagnosis is made and give all people the benefit of a positive treatment program.

Senility embarasses most of us, so we often shove out of heart and mind those whose thoughts and memories fall short of reality. We may no longer take them seriously as individuals, and we may freely talk about them in the third person almost as if they weren't there to hear us. By doing so, we strip them of whatever dignity they may have brought into old age and box them into an existence even more barren of joy and meaning. So, please remember if you are an advocate, you should make sure that the resident gets a positive treatment program, and doesn't get a "senile" label affixed across the forehead which basically implies *no help, no hope, no treatment.*

This practice must stop!

It is a simple, self-fulfilling prophecy that one often behaves and performs as institutionally expected. So if a label is stamped on a person's forehead, figuratively, of "senile" or "hopeless" it is self-explanatory that the practice is negative and a direct impediment to treatment and improvement.

A retired professor once said to me, "Thank heaven, you have taught your staff not to call me 'Pops,' or to pat me on the head like a dog." He went on, "And they don't treat me like a child or a dottering old man either...I feel accepted and treated as a responsible adult." Then he laughed and added, "... even though I am eccentric."

For those of you who remain skeptical about the effect of mislabeling or misdiagnosing someone, I would like to tell you a true heart-wrenching story about a lady named May. When we first purchased our facility, it became apparent that this lady, who was very infantile and regressed in her behavior, and very loud, active, and threatening to the staff, was in fact presenting a serious situation to be dealt with.

In the beginning, it was very difficult, because we were trying to accomplish so many things. It was very clear that this particular lady, who was only fifty-four years of age, and had been institutionalized for some twenty plus years, was in a pathetic circumstance, indeed. She would find staff members, and yell at them, put her arms around them from behind, frightening them, saying over and over, "Call Johnny, call Johnny!" Johnny was, of course, her husband who had remained at her side all of these years. He lived at home while May resided in various institutions.

My partner (also a registered nurse) and I observed her from time to time, and began paying special attention to her, trying to get to know her as a person *without any labels attached.* By the way, the original diagnosis was schizophrenia—chronic and undifferentiated type. It became apparent that she did, indeed, respond to positive reinforcement, and that her behavior could be modified by seeking her out *before* she came to get attention, and by expecting her to behave in a more appropriate adult-like manner. She did, in fact, respond favorably to these various treatment tools. Her mood swings were very dramatic, however, ranging from hysteria to seclusion. At times we would find her hiding in the closet. At other times, she would be screaming wildly in the halls. By now it's apparent to many of you who have studied psychology that this lady suffered from a manic-depressive disorder.

Fortunately, after much time and study, and appropriate charting to indicate these moods, we called in a psychiatrist who was willing to open May's case for re-testing. As a result, she was placed on lithium therapy, and within six weeks she was discharged home. Indeed, she had been given back her life. She and Johnny have been seen many times in town, walking hand-in-hand like two love birds recently reunited. This is a very touching story; it's *true,* and it *happened* in a *nursing home.*

This is only one true story, a dramatic one indeed, but there are thousands more such miracle stories inside the nursing home that you never hear or read about. Yes, I know there are horror stories too for which there is *no excuse.* I will tell you that, in my experience, these are far outnumbered by the day-to-day touching scenes and stories of love, friendship and bonding in the better nursing homes.

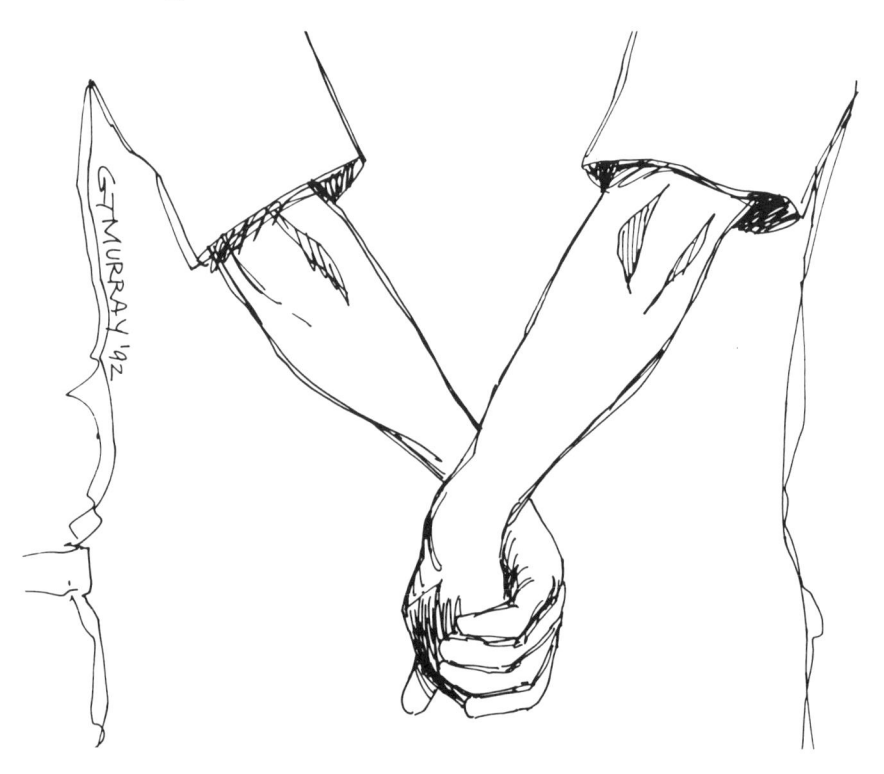

CHAPTER 7

Complaints and the Adjustment Period

Your concerns and comments as a family member or resident should be *welcomed* by the health-care center. At our nursing home, we always told people, "If you don't tell us, we can't correct it." Do not suffer and become upset in silence. Some complaints are valid; some are not. Some are merely misunderstandings that can be easily resolved with a little TLC. We have known a few residents who were absolutely delightful—pleasant, sociable, caring people—until their daughter arrived. Are these games people play? One lady told her daughter that we fed her "raw, uncooked noodles" and "raw bacon and lettuce" dinners. Obviously not true!

If the complaint is, "They lose all my clothes; I have nothing to wear," please remember that laundries in any large-scale operation are never as gentle as at home. My two teenage sons lost decent clothing—often in the washing machine in our own basement. We finally decided that the washing machine had "good taste," since it always left the grubbies intact.

If the resident has called the family member complaining, it may simply mean *"Come over here and see me!"* Now, if a brand-new dress or something of value is missing, see or call the administrator. He/she should try to track it down. One major problem in nursing homes is the "traveler" resident who picks up "pretty things." So, the missing article may not have been misdirected from the laundry, but may be found in another resident's room.

Another frequent complaint is, "They took my pudding, and I wanted it." The resident probably lifted it after dinner, and put it in a drawer to eat later. Some of the things that are lifted for later grow into a penicillin-like substance, and the stuff is obviously spoiled. The staff must monitor the drawers for these potential hazards. Often a good idea for the snacker or "hoarder" is to put a small refrigerator (dorm style) in the room. Then the "goodies" will at least be contained and at a proper temperature, although the situation still needs to be monitored, but better than in a drawer. If your mother is home and leaves crackers and cheese out to spoil, that's sad and too bad, but if she does it within the walls of a nursing home, that represents a serious violation for the facility.

Here is a list of the most frequent, usually unfounded complaints:

"I haven't seen a nurse in days!"

"No one brings me any food!"

"Some people around here get special treatment—not me!"

"They haven't cleaned my room all week!"

"I'm sick... so sick, and no one does anything about it!"

Any or all or some more imaginative statements may be heard. Generally—not always, but generally—this

Complaints and the Adjustment Period

translates to, "How come you haven't been here all week?" "How come you don't take me to live with you?" "How come you don't invite me for dinner... for church, for something—anything?" "Do you still care?" "Am I a part of the family?"

First and foremost is to listen to what is said. The facility should always check out complaints. *People should be believed* until proved otherwise. If a pattern has developed, then the facility can set up a behavior modification program to intervene. It is crucial that you the family member *listen* more than you respond. A simple, "Tell me all about it" shows you care and are willing to take the time to listen. Often there is a process of transference where your mother/father begins to depend less on you and more on the nursing facility staff. Special attachments take place during the initial adjustment period, and these will usually be long-term attachments. Please do not feel jealous or rejected. This is a good and necessary step towards adjustment and involvement within the facility. The bonds that do develop are strong, because the staff sees and works with, and gets to know, your mother/father on a daily basis.

Please remember that there is an *adjustment* period when a person enters a healthcare center. The unfamiliar sounds and people are very real whether is it a new house, apartment, a grand hotel or a healthcare facility. Once the resident is settled in, he/she should be taken on a grand tour to become familiar with the layout. This is a good opportunity to introduce the person to other residents and staff.

The family member should be *supportive,* be there when possible, and listen. You don't always *have to solve something.* Sometimes in our effort to solve things instantly at our center, we jumped the gun. One roomate in a double room complained, "I can't live with my roommate another minute...she's so obnoxious!" By the time we finished moving beds, furniture, and belongings, the two ladies were bosom buddies once again! Give the person time and space to transfer some needs over to the staff and other residents. We can choose our friends—not our family. The adjustment period may be as short as three days, or as long as two-plus weeks.

If the person is entering the healthcare center for an extended stay, together with the adjustment period, there will be a natural, grieving stage. Any loss causes mourning. Allow the person to talk, you just listen. Allow the person to cry—if she needs to—and just *be there*. This is a transitional period, and we as children or the spouse, should not panic and feed negatively into this normal pattern. Should the new resident be the spouse (could be fifty plus years) and maybe even a long-term caregiver, it can be especially traumatic to no longer feel needed. In this situation, the facility should encourage the former caregiver to share all the special little things, and to remain a vital part of the care plan, day to day. This spouse is not about to immediately trust the staff. It should be as a joint/team effort with the spouse as a member *on* the inside, *not* as an outsider.

The healthcare center should have qualified staff members who will be able to lighten the adjustment period, so please do not hesitate to ask for help; psychological hurt can be as painful as a physical wound. Both problems can fester if ignored. The best facilities will make frequent contact with you to see how you feel "things are going." As mentioned in the first paragraph, please tell them what's on your mind, as well as any concerns or worries you may have.

CHAPTER 8

The Nursing Home Industry—A Bad Rap

The nursing home industry itself is generally good, and yet the stigma remains. Nursing homes often remain at the top of the loser's list— "a last resort," "a perilous place," "a cesspool," "a stinky, miserable, depressing graveyard!" "Why?" you ask. Much of nursing homes' maligned image and stigma are the result of abuses of the past, the greed factor, and the absence of sound, enforceable regulations in the early days.

However, increased awareness, concern, and devotion by industry and advocacy groups required the nursing home industry to become better regulated, some say second only to nuclear energy. Some regulations remain "paper" oriented which take away from "people" priorities, though most are good and necessary. Certainly, more highly educated, caring professionals are aimed towards excellence. The truth is, you will have more difficulty in seeking to resolve a "lemon" car warranty than you will encounter in solving a problem in a sub-standard nursing home. To be sure, there are still a few nursing homes that do not deserve to continue in their present mode, but happily their number is dwindling. The facilities doing a good job do enjoy an enhanced, positive image. However, sensationalistic horror stories continue to make the news. The good, kind, positive, inspirational, warm-fuzzy stuff doesn't. One horror story wipes out *thousands* of loving, caring, wonderful, touching miracle stories. Here is an example I know to be factual, because it happened at a facility I know. The nursing home had rented limos to take some of the residents to a chicken barbecue in our community. One of the resident council members called the local newspaper to suggest that they cover this event with a story and perhaps a picture. The residents were so excited and thrilled over the thought of riding in a limo. "What to wear?," "I can't wait to tell my family"... "Wow!" There was excitement in the air. Most of the older adults have always been excessively frugal (by today's standards), and this was a "big deal"—a first, an event!

The media did not find it interesting. Yet, if there had been a minor trash fire in a utility room—no damage, no threat, no problem—don't you know that would have been considered newsworthy, and would have probably appeared on the front page of some newspaper. Biased news?—of course. We all recognize the impact that the media exercises on major events— such as presidential elections and world happenings. I believe they have a responsibility to write about the good stuff too. Think of it—headlines of joyful, wonderful, and good news! How else can we have the truth? I think it's analogous to the press presentation of today's teenagers. One would assume that most of them are on drugs, alcohol, and are sexually promiscuous. You know what an unfair and dangerous assumption that is, much

The Nursing Home Industry—A Bad Rap

as the "horror" stories about nursing homes grab the headlines and disseminate adverse generalizations over the entire industry. Maybe if the stories were uplifting, we would all be inspired to have a better day. In fairness, I have to say that our local media did cover lots of "good things" and it helped counteract the negative stigma enormously.

I write this by way of background, to hopefully assist you to be open-minded, and not be blinded by media sensationalism—any more than you would be blinded by a glistening chandelier in choosing a nursing home. Whether it be a retirement center, a hospital-based, long-term care unit or a homecare agency, they each need and desire your business. After all, each is—or certainly should be—in the business of service. Serving the needs of *individuals* must be the essence of their existence. Of course, the word *service* has

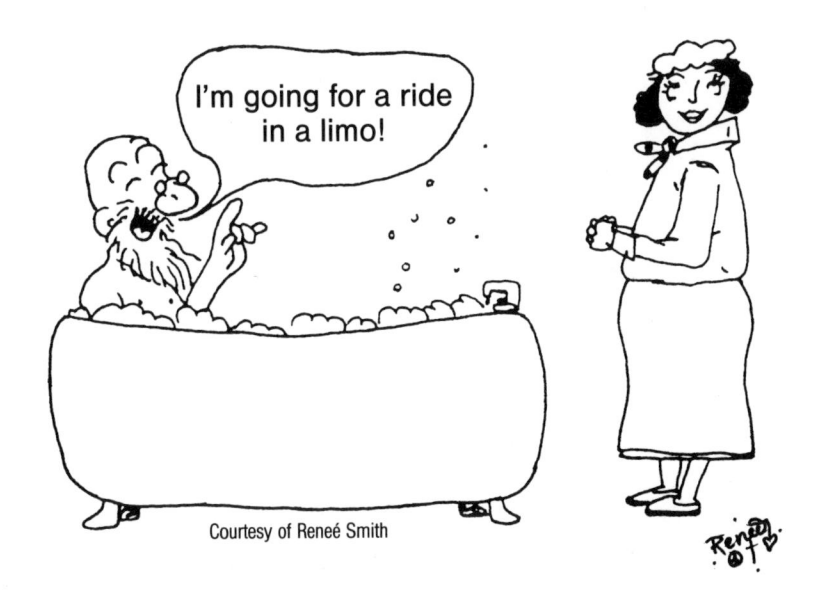

I'm going for a ride in a limo!

Courtesy of Reneé Smith

become a popular media-hype word. "Service is Our Business" is used everywhere from car repair shops to "The Hospital with a Heart." That seems absurd, because we already expect hospitals and nursing care centers to do it "from the heart." In many cases, I have found the very people who will say to the staff at the nursing home, "I love it here; I love the attention; I love having so many friends; I love all the activities; I'm excited about life again!" somehow find it almost impossible to say those things to family members. It's almost a self-fulfilling prophecy kind of thing. If the family has somehow gotten the message to Mother, "Oh God, how terrible we feel that we had to send you to the nursing home. We just feel awful about it. We will forever be sorry!" Then somehow the person (resident) feels as if that level of guilt on the part of the family has to be sustained. I read in Barbara Johnson's book titled *Stick A Geranium in Your Hat and Be Happy,* "My mother is a travel agent for guilt trips." Therefore, it then becomes very difficult for the resident to upset the family by saying, "Hey, this is great!" I have heard this scenario played out many times, and I believe it needs to be mentioned.

CHAPTER 9

Predictions for the Industry

"Please send me to the nursing home," mother said as she was barely coming out from under the anesthesia following hip prosthesis surgery. What to do but abide by her wishes! After all, she had always taken care of me—been there for me—and now I find myself in the "mother mode" for my own mother! Ah, you say, science fiction at its best! If only it could be like that; mother *asking* to go to a nursing home. As we all know, what occurs in reality is, "I'll come back and haunt you if you *ever* send me to the nursing home" or, "I'd rather die!" In reality the "F" word (FEAR) has been indelibly implanted in many brains, and surfaces each time a new sensationalistic, horror story about nursing homes hits the front page. "See, I keep telling you how terrible they are... don't ever send me there." This gives rise to the "G" word (GUILT) for the family.

All of you who watched the 20/20 TV edition recently concerning nursing homes neglecting residents relate to this profound, very real fear older people have of nursing homes. What was shown on this documentary was scandalous and sickening. Had I the power, I would have closed those disgraceful facilities and moved all those people to another facility like the ones shown in the introduction of the telecast. You know now who to call for immediate help to assist you should you find yourself or a loved one in this kind of facility. However, money, as in federal and state Medicaid funds allocated to nursing home care, is a real problem; it needs to be looked at realistically in terms of our society's commitment to the care of the elderly.

If it costs fifty to sixty dollars plus per night for a motel room, why would the government believe that a nursing home resident can be cared for at a lesser price than a motel rate? Does the motel provide around-the-clock nursing care and all meals? All the new regulations, which are good and necessary, require increased staffing and programs among other things, which obviously cost the facilities more. So it can and does become a Catch 22 situation, and this is intolerable. People who don't have sufficient funds, or who spend down all of their assets on medical and nursing home care deserve the same treatment, respect, and dignity accorded the private-pay residents. Maybe that's idealistic but surely our government will prioritize the needs of our senior citizens. Maybe it is time for Medicare to include long-term care provisions, as well as a more equitable form of reimbursement to healthcare facilities who *do* provide excellent care.

Many of you have read the story about a lady named Ethel who died, and many of her friends threw a party, because she would *never* have to go to a nursing home. Most older people feel exactly the same way: "Say anything, go anywhere, do anything, but please *never* put me in a nursing home!" It is a statement based on fear and all the sensationalistic horror stories. You know what? They truly are scared to death, because all they have heard is the bad propaganda. All of this "bad" press is extremely harmful to the person who is facing this decision.

There *are* good, caring facilities out there. Now that I am no longer an owner of a healthcare center, I can say these things with credibility. In the past, some might have said, "Well sure, she feels that way; she owns a nursing home. Of course she would have nice things to say about healthcare centers!" It has been my contention for years that those healthcare facilities which don't measure up to standards and provide quality care *ought to be closed.* I don't know why this doesn't occur oftener because there are more and more advocacy groups such as AARP, the Area Agency on Aging, and the Ombudsman Program out there watching and observing, assuring that the proper kind of care is delivered. Also the federal and state licensure accreditation surveys assure standards are being met, and these are public records. With increased competition and availability, *you should not have to accept or reside in a substandard facility.*

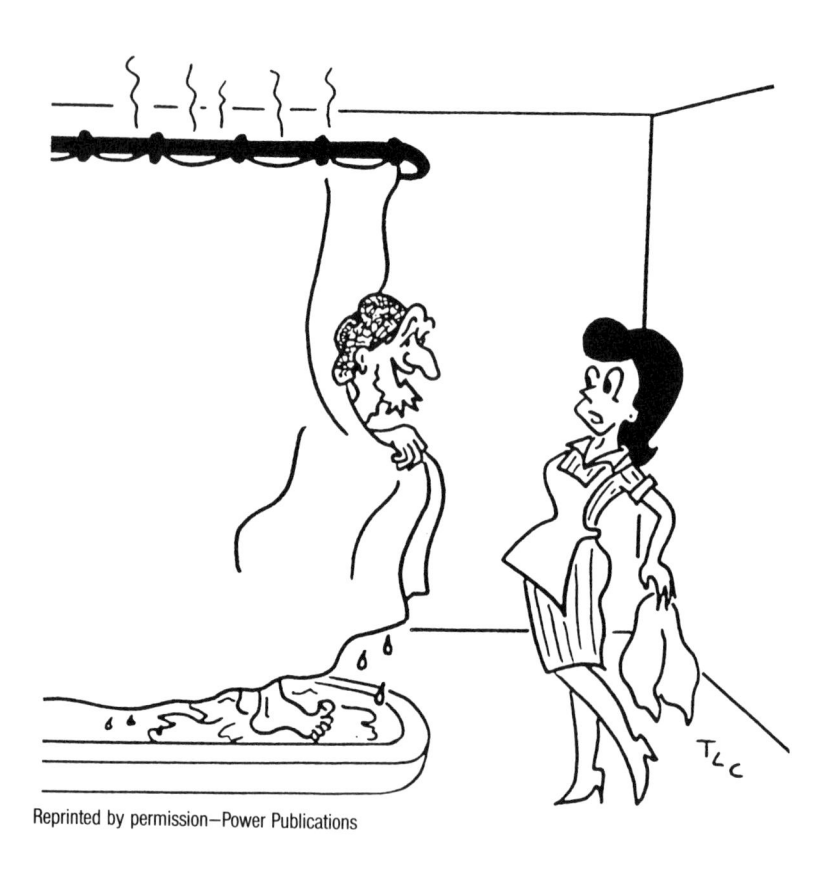

"Care to join me?"

---

*Age is a state of mind,
don't ask me what state I'm in!*

CHAPTER 10

Conclusion

I sincerely hope this book has been helpful to you, especially to the older person who lives in fear of the nursing home and to the families who agonize in guilt and indecision for lack of "how to choose and what to do."

My need to share my thoughts, ideals, and positive experiences was quite simply something I wanted to do on a personal level.

On the professional level, naturally I hope the industry people will continue their quest to achieve the *best* status. Should any nursing homes take some suggestions or ideas from this writing, I would be honored. Those facilities that are in the Best of the Best category could probably have added another whole dimension to this presentation. Hats off, praise to them and God bless. Those homes that *don't* measure up and *don't* even try...well, people will not beat a path to their door. They may, however, form a line that leads to the exit, and they should NOW.

To recap: You really are in charge and you have the ability to make informed decisions with love, care and

concern. If you find yourself needing to choose a nursing home, you can make the right choices based on careful visitation, analysis, and knowledge of what to look for by:
What is *seen* with your own eyes
Felt in your heart
Known by your instincts.

I have to restate the caution not to be dazzled by the glitzy brochures, ice cream parlors, and chandeliers, but to focus primarily on the *human factor* operating within. You now know how to look with confidence for that *people oriented* place where it's routine to break routine, so as to give you personalized attention. A place where you will be treated with respect and "handled with care" and dignity, because you deserve it. You cannot expect to find perfection, but you can find the right place for you. It will show itself when you feel a comfortable peace. We all know that love is hard to define, but we certainly *know* it when we find it.

Fortunately, I seem to find love everywhere. Perhaps because I choose to look for it, nurture it and treasure it. Even though I am an incurable optimist and guilty of accentuating the positive, I am also keenly aware of the negative stigma surrounding the nursing home issue. By most accounts, the nursing home dilemma is perceived as a dreaded, feared, excruciatingly painful, guilt-laden process. I hope this book has helped to dispel some myths, preconceived notions and to unclog some of the hardening of the negative attitudes.

Those of you who have made the effort to read this book and do your homework are to be congratulated. You obviously want the knowledge and perspective to do the right thing and choose among the best because *you do care deeply.*

Conclusion

In closing, I want to THANK YOU for caring and wish for you peace and love as you go forth to make the Right Choices.

*The best
and most beautiful
things in the world
cannot be seen,
nor touched...
but are felt
in the heart.*

         Helen Keller

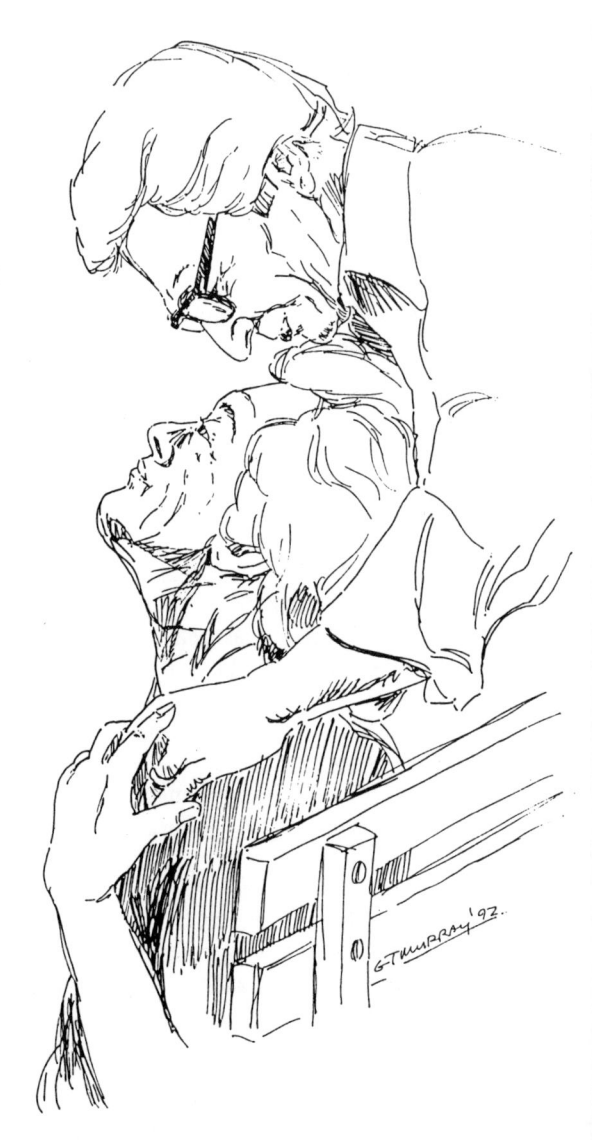

There is a poem titled "Don't Be Fooled By Me". It should be "must reading" for all healthcare providers. The poem is printed here, because it very eloquently points out the need to be recognized and to be thought of as a special, unique individual.

Don't Be Fooled By Me

Don't be fooled by me, don't be fooled by the face I wear.
For I wear a Thousand Masks, masks that I'm afraid to take off, and none of them is me.
Pretending is an art that's second nature with me, but don't be fooled, for God's sake.
Don't be fooled.

I give the impression that I'm secure, that all is sunny and unruffled with me.
Within as well as without, that confidence is my name and coolness is my game.
That the water's calm and I'm in command, and that I need no one.
But don't believe me, please.

My surface may seem smooth, but my surface is my mask.
Beneath this lies no complacence.
Beneath dwells the real me in confusion, in fear, and aloneness.
But I hide this. I don't want anyone to know it.
I panic at the thought of my weakness and fear of being exposed.
That's why I frantically create a mask to hide behind, a nonchalant, sophisticated facade,
To help me pretend, to shield me from the glance that knows.
But such a glance is precisely my salvation. My only salvation.
And I know it.

That is, if it's followed by acceptance, if it's followed by love.
It's the only thing that will assure me of what I can't assure myself,
That I am worth something.
But I don't tell you this. I don't dare.
I'm afraid to.
I'm afraid that your glance will not be followed by acceptance and love.
I'm afraid that you'll think less of me, that you'll laugh at me.
Your laugh would kill me.
I'm afraid that deep down I'm nothing, that I'm no good and you will see this and reject me.
So, I play the game, my desperate game, with a facade of assurance without
And a trembling child within.
And so begins the parade of masks.
And my life becomes a front.

I idly chatter to you in suave tones of surface talk.
I tell you everything that is really nothing and nothing of what's everything.
Of what's crying within me; so when I'm going through my routine, do not be fooled by what I'm saying. Please *listen carefully* and try *to hear what I am not saying,*
What I'd like to be able to say, what, *for survival,* I need *to say,* but what *I can't say.*

Introspective Poem

I dislike hiding. Honestly! I dislike
the superficial game I'm playing,
the phony game.
I'd really like to be genuine and
spontaneous, and me—but you've
got to help me.
You've got to hold out your hand,
even when that's the last thing
I seem to want.
Only you can wipe away from my
eyes the blank stare of
breathing death.

Only you can call me into aliveness.
Each time you're *kind* and *gentle*
and *encouraging,*
Each time *you try to understand*
because you really care,
My heart begins to grow wings,
very small wings, very feeble
wings, but wings.
With your sensitivity and sympathy,
and your power of understanding,
You can breathe life into me.
I want *you to know that.*

I want you to know how important
you are to me.
How you can be the creator of the
person that is me if you choose to.
Please, choose to.
You alone can break down the wall
behind which I tremble.
You alone can remove my mask.
You alone can release me from my
shadow-world of panic and
uncertainty from my lonely person.
Do not pass me by. Please . . .
do not pass me by.

It will not be easy for you.
A long conviction of worthlessness
builds strong walls.
The nearer you approach me, the
blinder I strike back.
I fight against the very thing I
cry out for.
But I am told that love is stronger
than walls, and in this lies my hope.
Please try to beat down those walls
with firm hands, but with
gentle hands.
For a child is very sensitive.
Who am I, you may wonder. I am
someone you know very well.
For I am *every man* you meet.
And I am *every woman* you meet.

Anonymous

Suggested Reading
(Available information sources)

American Association of Retired Persons (AARP)
601 E. Street, N.W.
Washington, D.C. 20049
Available booklets pertaining to nursing homes:
  Nursing Home Life (D-13063)
  Tomorrow's Choices (D-13479)
  Establishing a Nursing Home Community Council (D-13385)

U.S. Department of Health and Human Services
Health Care Financing Administration
6325 Security Boulevard
Baltimore, Maryland 21207
Helpful booklets that are available:
  Guide to Choosing a Nursing Home Pub. No. HCFA-02174
  Medicare Q & A
  The Medicare Handbook
  Guide to Health Insurance for People with Medicare (507-X)
  Medicare and Coordinated Care Plans (509-X)
  Medicare Hospice Benefits (508-X)

Federal Council on the Aging (FCA)
HEW North, Room 4260
330 Independence Avenue, S.W.
Washington, D.C. 20201

National Council of Senior Citizens (NCSC)
925 15th St., N.W.
Washington, D.C. 20005

The National Council on the Aging, Inc. (NCOA)
600 Maryland Avenue, S.W.
West Wing 100
Washington, D.C. 20024

I Work in a Home Full of Love

Welcome to our nursing home; just walk right in, don't be afraid or hesitate. This is a nursing home full of love and caring. I work here.

Just start down the hallways, we have two north and south wings with a dining room between. Notice the people as you walk along—smile! We are very busy here working, you see, to make things even better for our residents. Improvement. Great. We wash and we clean, we feed those who need. We walk and we talk to whoever we take care of.

Hope is essential as so is their space. We have a lot of love here and so we all give. I work as a rehab aide in a nursing home. I ambulate all residents who can walk. I apply splints and perform range-of-motion too. I also work with physical therapists. In this way, I am learning more to help our residents. My job helps decrease discomfort by movement. This is an example of a caring nursing home. I have the main function of one employee just to ambulate and do range-of-motion for the residents in my care to help their circulation, lower their number of contractures, and help their self-esteem. We all care.

Taking great pride in any task we do, whether it be bathing, feeding, walking, shows we care. We work as a team. The residents shine. So we shine with them.

Hope is very hard for residents in a nursing home; therefore, I feel it is very important to them to have trust and confidence in us as nursing home employees. We all try to make our nursing home as close to a family unit as we can for our residents, but at the same time we do not enter their time or space, unless we are welcome. We wait and respect.

I believe each employee in a nursing home has to reach out and make each resident an extension of his/her own family with love, caring, and respect.

We care and do love.

Betty Shaffer, QMA

I Care:
I Work in a Nursing Home

I work in a nursing home because I care. I chose nursing not really knowing what to expect from it. I have experienced and shared the joys, tears, some of their hopes and dreams and I feel as if I belong to each and every one of those sweet people. I never dreamed the rewards of nursing were so great. I love and care for each of my residents here. The little things I do for them day-by-day, like helping to feed them when their hands are too shaky to hold a spoon, or when I help bathe them or tie their shoes when they aren't able.

Things in everyday life we do are chores for them. I give them a little encouragement to keep trying and a smile or a hug lets me know they appreciate what I do for them. It's not just a job to me, it's a way of life. I love what I do and I'm good at it.

I put a lot into working here, but I get much more in return than I ever thought. I strongly believe it takes a special kind of person to work in a nursing home. You have to care for and love our residents like they were family. Not that I am a special person in any way, but the feelings I get from helping and caring for them are special and make it all worthwhile. To treat them with the respect and dignity they deserve, you must have feeling and compassion to give of yourself and not ask for anything in return but a smile.

There is a special look in their eyes even though they can't say your name. But I know in my heart they care and love me as much as I love them. I listen to them talk about yesteryears, not only with my ears but with my heart. I am their friend, I talk to them, but I am also their family. To some I am the only family they have, so I enjoy sharing my family with them.

I am very honored and proud to be a part of this nursing home. The years here have taught me a lot. I wouldn't give any of it up; I'm doing something worthwhile and I'm proud of my job. The rewards of working in a nursing home are heaven sent. No, I'm not talking about money, it's the way I feel about helping others—people who need me and depend on me. Everyone should experience working in a nursing home at least one time in their lives. I guess that's why God gave me such a big heart. I grow to love and treasure each and every person in a different way. I have learned from them, I feel I have made a difference in some of their lives, and they make a big difference in my life also. I know I need them as much as they need me. I have gotten much more in return than I could ever give. I know when I leave at the end of the day, I have done a good job. I can rest with that.

Ina Henke, QMA

I Understand What Caring Is

It all started a few years ago when I decided to get a part-time job. If anyone would have told me it was going to be a loving, caring and sharing experience, I probably would have said, "Oh, sure!"

I worked in a factory for sixteen years, I liked my job, but of course it was just a job. I quit to stay home with my daughter until she started school.

A job became available in my town. It was in a nursing home. I applied for the job and was hired on as a part-time housekeeper. My very first day was my orientation. I sat through what seemed like a long two hours of a lot of rules. When it was over I went home that day and began to think of what I had just listened to. I asked myself: Do we really have to care that much? I'm hiring in to clean rooms and toilets. A lot of orientation was on safety and fire rules. Well, of course we always had safety rules in the factory, but never a fire drill or test on them. It was pretty much everyone for himself. I asked myself again, "Do I really have to care that much?"

I went to sleep that night still thinking about the responsibility I would have and wondering if it was going to be worth it; after all, I was going to be a housekeeper.

It was my first day and it all started to make sense. The day I walked in the door and down the hallway, someone greeted me with a smile and said, "Good morning, dear, how are you?" Here was a beautiful lady who didn't even know me asking me how I was. Was this the caring? As the days went by, my job seemed to grow on me. I've always considered myself a loving, caring person but working in a nursing home as the years roll by has let me understand the meaning of caring.

The residents are like family. I've cried with them, cried for them, and they have also helped me through some rough times. I've made a lot of close friends. I really don't know of any job I could have where I get up every day knowing that I'm appreciated. Every day the "pleases" and "thank yous" I get from my job are enough to keep me coming back for more.

Yes, I really do care and every day at some point I think back to that orientation and ask again, "Do I really have to care that much?" No, I don't *have* to. I *want* to!

I'm a full-time housekeeper now; I've learned a lot and still learning every day. It's been a rewarding experience. I wish everyone could be as lucky as I've been to be part of a nursing home staff.

Onward to another year of loving, caring, and lots of smiles.

Leesa Price, Housekeeper

Caring that People are Happy

A resident enters a nursing home because he or she needs a form of assistance with daily functions. Over the last twelve years I have been at the nursing home as a healthcare provider.

My goal each day is to do my best to keep each resident healthy, physically active, mentally alert, socially acceptable, and a happy individual. I care that each resident has a clean, temperature-controlled environment, comfortable clothing, proper medical care, "tasty" nutritional food and drink. I care that each has a social life as he is accustomed and desires. Contacts outside the facility are very important, such as visitors, clubs, religious affiliation, transportation to and from, access to a private phone for personal use. I care that the resident continues learning experiences, mental stimulation, and hobbies of his desires.

All of the above should be employed for each resident as he or she desires. I want to be part of ensuring that the resident has these opportunities each day.

No, even though this is what I want for each resident, I, as one health caregiver, cannot provide it all to all residents. But I can work with a caring team of workers and find the proper person to assist in all these actions. Just because the resident has changed shelter structures does not mean he or she must behave in a changed manner. I want for each resident the right to be his or her own individual self.

The resident entered the nursing home for a little assistance. I enter the nursing home to provide the most individualistic, loving assistance that I as one caregiver can provide. I truly care that humans who need assistance with daily functions should have quality living for the remainder of their lives.

I care: I work in a nursing home.

Mary E. Morris, Activity Director

Visitation Check List

Visitation Check List

APPEARANCE

1. Exterior
What is your first impression? Are the grounds well maintained and attractive (shrubs, flowers, litter free, etc.)?
☐ Yes ☐ No

Is there a patio area with outdoor seating? ☐ Yes ☐ No

Is there adequate parking? ☐ Yes ☐ No

2. Interior
General state of *cleanliness* (without being sterile and institutional) _____

Odor free? ☐ Yes ☐ No

Floors? ☐ Good ☐ Average ☐ Poor

Dining/lounge rooms, kitchen, hallways?
☐ Good ☐ Average ☐ Poor

Non-institutional "feel" or *appearance* (are there wall hangings, plants, pictures and color)?
☐ Good ☐ Average ☐ Poor

3. Residents' Rooms
Most important: Does it appear "lived-in", "home-like"? Are personal effects displayed—art and craft work, pictures on walls, cards displayed, a favorite chair or other pieces to *personalize* the room?
☐ Good ☐ Average ☐ Poor ☐ None

Private bathroom and bathing facilities?
☐ Good ☐ Average ☐ Poor ☐ None

Visitation Check List

Lighting for reading, work; desk space for doing personal business?
☐ Good ☐ Average ☐ Poor ☐ None

Closet/drawer/storage space?
☐ Good ☐ Average ☐ Poor ☐ None

4. Environment—Atmosphere

Try to speak with the residents and/or family members.

Do you **feel** and sense a *caring* atmosphere?
☐ Yes ☐ No

Does the facility appear "active and alive"?
☐ Yes ☐ No

Is there a sense of something happening, some noise?
☐ Yes ☐ No

Do the residents appear content and happy?
☐ Yes ☐ No

Do the residents seem to be *respectfully* and *affectionately* cared for and about?
☐ Yes ☐ No

5. Environment—Physical Plant

Does the facility practice good safety/cleanliness techniques?
☐ Yes ☐ No

Are the hallways unobstructed and well lighted with non-slip floors?
☐ Yes ☐ No

Does the facility have a sprinkler system, disaster drills, etc.?
☐ Yes ☐ No

6. Dining Rooms and
7. Lounges

Conducive to conversation and home like (are people facing each other, involved with each other, or are all chairs lined up in a row)?

☐ Good ☐ Average ☐ Poor

Well lighted, tablecloths, flowers, etc. on tables?

☐ Good ☐ Average ☐ Poor ☐ None

8. Staff Involvement

Observe attitudes of the staff. What kind of communication is going on?

☐ Good ☐ Average ☐ Poor ☐ None

Do they take time for the "little things" that are so important (a hug, a smile, friendly, warm communication)?

☐ Yes ☐ No

Adequate in numbers?
(Check response to calls for assistance.)

☐ Yes ☐ No

Generally happy in their work (smiling and talking with residents)?

☐ Yes ☐ No

9. Residents' Rights

Most Important: Do you sense and see a high priority regarding dignity, quality, and enhancement of life?

☐ Yes ☐ No

Ask to see and *read* the Residents' Rights statements.

Are children/grandchildren welcome and invited to share in activities and programs?

☐ Yes ☐ No

Are family members encouraged to remain fully and actively involved in the care program and plan?
☐ Yes ☐ No

Are *individuality* and *choices encouraged* (not simply allowed but encouraged)?
☐ Yes ☐ No

Does staff respect privacy (doors closed when treatments and care given, etc.)?
☐ Yes ☐ No

Are the residents encouraged to do their *own thing* if able (some may wish to stay up for the Late Show and some may wish to have coffee at 6:00 a.m.)?
☐ Yes ☐ No

Medical, Nursing and Care Needs
Professional licensed nurses on duty 24 hours per day around the clock? Do they make rounds with kindness and compassion?
☐ Yes ☐ No

How does the facility handle medical emergencies? _____

_____

Does a podiatrist, dentist, etc. come see residents at the facility?
☐ Yes ☐ No

Ratio of professional nurses and aides _____

10. Adult Day Care, Respite Care, Home Health Care

What services are provided? What is the cost per hour/day? What is included in the program?

_____
_____
_____

11. Restoration and Rehabilitation

Is there an active exercise program; are therapists available?

☐ Good   ☐ Average   ☐ Poor   ☐ None

What is the restraint policy? _____
_____

Preventative Care

Are residents encouraged to remain as independent as possible, encouraged to walk, etc.?

☐ Yes   ☐ No

If the resident so desires and is capable, is there a plan of care to return the resident home or to a less expensive level of care?

☐ Yes   ☐ No

12. Observe the Residents

Do they appear clean and well groomed?

☐ Good   ☐ Average   ☐ Poor

Is there a beauty/barber shop in the facility?

☐ Yes   ☐ No

Are they dressed appropriately?

☐ Good   ☐ Average   ☐ Poor

Observe the condition of hair, nails, eyeglasses, etc.

☐ Good   ☐ Average   ☐ Poor

Visitation Check List

13. Resident Council
Is it active and involved in the decision making process?
☐ Good ☐ Average ☐ Poor ☐ None

14. Dietary
Ask about special diets.

Is the weekly menu posted? ☐ Yes ☐ No

Are selections, choices, needs and preferences honored?
☐ Yes ☐ No

Is the kitchen sanitary and orderly?
☐ Good ☐ Average ☐ Poor

Observe a meal (eat a meal if possible).
☐ Good ☐ Average ☐ Poor

15. Spiritual Needs
Are church services, Bible study, etc. offered?
☐ Good ☐ Average ☐ Poor

16. Activities/Social Services
Ask to see the monthly calendar of events.

What is happening while you are there? _____

Are the activities varied and diversified to meet the needs of all?
☐ Good ☐ Average ☐ Poor

Are there classes offered for mental/intellectual stimulation?
☐ Good ☐ Average ☐ Poor ☐ None

What is the involvement with the community?
☐ Good ☐ Average ☐ Poor ☐ None

Is the family involved and their valuable input solicited? (Is there a family council?)
☐ Yes ☐ No

Are outings with family, friends and other residents encouraged (such as shopping trips, concerts, etc.)?
☐ Yes ☐ No

17. Financial/Levels of Care Provided

What is the actual cost per day/month? _____

Are there any additional costs (laundry, level of care, beauty shop, etc.)?
☐ Yes ☐ No

Does the dailty rate go up if care needs increase?
☐ Yes ☐ No

Medicare/Medicaid assistance program available (what happens when private money is exhausted)?
☐ Yes ☐ No

Is the facility Medicare/Medicaid certified?
☐ Yes ☐ No

MOST IMPORTANT

Do you feel the *sincerity* and *caring* attitude of the staff?
☐ Yes ☐ No

Do *people* come first? ☐ Yes ☐ No

Do you feel *confidence* and *trust*? ☐ Yes ☐ No

Will *your* involvement and input be *valued* and *encouraged*?
☐ Yes ☐ No

*Work with the facility. Be part of the team.
Get and stay involved.*

Visitation Check List

NOTES

Copyright © 1992 by Lynn Smith, R.N.